SEP 25 2013

Warmed by Windchill

MAR 17 2015

Middleton
7425 Hub
Middleton, WI 53562
D0720867

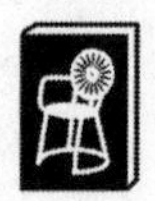

Terrace Books, a trade imprint of the University of Wisconsin Press, takes its name from the Memorial Union Terrace, located at the University of Wisconsin–Madison. Since its inception in 1907, the Wisconsin Union has provided a venue for students, faculty, staff, and alumni to debate art, music, politics, and the issues of the day. It is a place where theater, music, drama, literature, dance, outdoor activities, and major speakers are made available to the campus and the community. To learn more about the Union, visit www.union.wisc.edu.

Warmed by Windchill

A Tiny Colt's Fight for Life

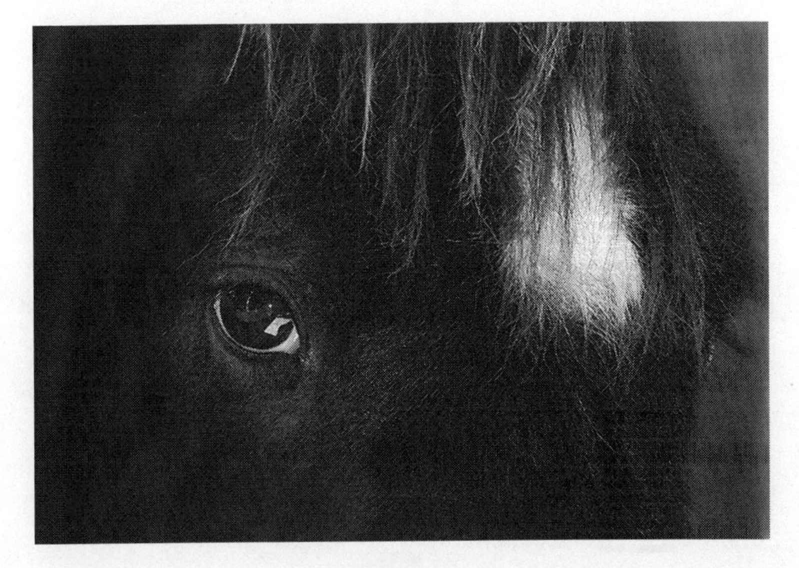

Jeffrey L. Tucker

TERRACE BOOKS
A trade imprint of the University of Wisconsin Press

Terrace Books
A trade imprint of the University of Wisconsin Press
1930 Monroe Street, 3rd Floor
Madison, Wisconsin 53711-2059
uwpress.wisc.edu

3 Henrietta Street
London WC2E 8LU, England
eurospanbookstore.com

Copyright © 2013 by Jeffrey L. Tucker
All rights reserved. No part of this publication may be reproduced, stored in a retrieval system, or transmitted, in any format or by any means, digital, electronic, mechanical, photocopying, recording, or otherwise, or conveyed via the Internet or a website without written permission of the University of Wisconsin Press, except in the case of brief quotations embedded in critical articles and reviews.

Printed in the United States of America

Library of Congress Cataloging-in-Publication Data

Tucker, Jeffrey L.
Warmed by Windchill: a tiny colt's fight for life / Jeffrey L. Tucker.
p. cm.
Includes bibliographical references.
ISBN 978-0-299-29404-5 (pbk.: alk. paper)
ISBN 978-0-299-29403-8 (e-book)
1. Horses—Wisconsin. 2. Animal rescue—Wisconsin. I. Title.
HV4749.T83 2013
636.1'0709775II—dc23
2013007168

The cover photograph is copyrighted by the Windchill Legacy Ltd. (thewindchilllegacy.org), the nonprofit organization created by Windchill's caregivers as a result of his plight. The Windchill Legacy addresses equine neglect, abuse, and overpopulation, and it educates the public about these issues while supporting equine rescues. The photo is the group's logo and is used here with the express permission of the Windchill Legacy Ltd. Board of Directors.

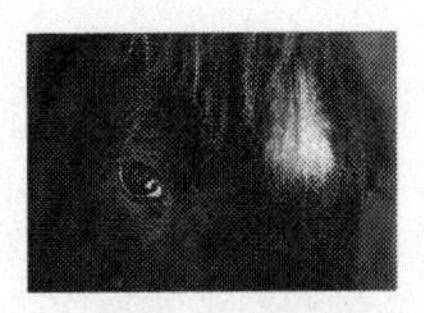

This book is dedicated to
those with the desire to help the innocent,
to
the quietly courageous who race to the aid of those in need—
living beings without a voice or ability to help themselves.

This book is dedicated to
those who stand up for what they believe is right—
not for any recognition, but purely because it's the right thing to do.

More than likely right now somewhere near you is a person keeping vigil. Maybe they're alone trying to care for a sick loved one night and day. Maybe they're a team of caring volunteers scrambling to find the time and resources to heal a terribly hurt animal.

It's to their spirit and devotion I dedicate this book.

One step at a time, one being at a time, they are quietly changing the world.

Contents

Foreword

CAROLYN L. STULL, PHD

Horses are one of the most incredible animals that have intertwined my life. As a very young girl, I read a small old book that my mother placed in my bedroom. That book was *Black Beauty*. I spent my waking hours at the local stable with both human and equine friends. My parents soon bought me a kind and lovely blue-roan mare, Dolly, who received my constant attention and admiration. I spent hours reading books and magazines absorbing information on how to make her look pretty and feed and care for her. I tirelessly trained her for riding with friends and at local competitions.

What truly fascinated me about Dolly was trying to understand what she was thinking or how she perceived her own little world, especially the people in it. I think most people who love animals and have pets would like to know what they're thinking.

When I left for college, Dolly came with me. The campus had stables, and I was not about to go months without her. In school I pursued studies on all the subjects that pertained to horse care and behavior and eventually earned a doctoral degree. On a cold and snowy day soon after graduation, I accepted a job at the University of California–Davis in the area of animal welfare. In time I received funding for a research project examining refeeding programs for horses that were starved.

Emaciated horses were brought from Mexico to the campus to be used as subjects for testing the different types of feed. It was the most emotionally exhausting research project: balancing the fact that eight starved horses were so easily acquired, there was a distinct split among my fellow faculty members on their support of my efforts, and the reality that several horses were euthanized during the early studies. The plus side is that the information gleaned from these studies to help refeed starved and neglected horses has been circulated around the world, now often accessed with the click of a search button on the Internet.

That is exactly how I connected with Kathi Davis and Jeff Tucker in Wisconsin concerning their rescue of a little colt they named Windchill. An e-mail was sent asking me about diet and care for this extremely weak and emaciated colt. I immediately responded giving them my best scientific approach to Windchill's feeding plan, which included offering the forage alfalfa. But I also knew that the rehabilitation of Windchill would require many daily decisions by Kathi and Jeff and that their physical and emotional energy would need to be strong and relentless.

Both Kathi and Jeff should be commended for their coordinated integration and persistent efforts during this extraordinary journey of uncertainty. Their story, *Warmed by Windchill*, reflects their total commitment and loyalty to the welfare of any horse, as well as their unique gift to align themselves with the thoughts and perceptions of one very cold and hungry colt. The story is inspirational to those who simply admire or provide lifelong care for any "incredible" horse.

Dr. Carolyn L. Stull is a Cooperative Extension Specialist in the School of Veterinary Medicine at the University of California–Davis. Her educational program focuses on the well-being of agricultural animals in local communities, while her research interests include the development of dietary programs for starved and healthy horses, the study of transportation stress, and the care and outcome of unwanted horses in society.

Warmed by Windchill

Prologue

Kathi was back in a hurry.

"We need to do something about that horse," she said, racing into the house. "It doesn't have more than a couple hours." And with those few words, our quiet Saturday went from zero to ninety, and our lives took a turn I'm still learning how to maneuver.

The winter of 2007–8 was an especially harsh one in northwestern Wisconsin. Pounded by snow in December, brutal cold followed in February. It was one of the coldest winters in decades. Even the most rugged and stoic of our lifelong residents were talking about it.

Shivering the second I slipped outside to do chores, I would hurry back inside as soon as I finished them and watch the wind and snow from the comfort of a living room heated by a roaring fire. But that was no longer the case nine days into February. Starting on that Saturday and for twenty days thereafter, almost all of my waking hours traded a warm house for a cold horse barn. The reason would forever change my life.

Until this experience, I assumed people believed as I did about certain things. I can accept we have different views on politics, where to live, the foods we like, God, and religion. I could not accept others would believe abuse of any kind was acceptable, whether it be children, pets, or partners. And as the owner of a horse farm, I always thought no one would willfully abuse or neglect something so beautiful, so majestic, as a horse, right?

I was wrong.

1

The Orange Sled

The wind started before dawn. Hearing it from beneath the comfort of warm blankets did not make the idea of getting out of bed a good one. But life on a horse farm near Lake Superior in February means animals need to be checked, ice on top of the water tanks needs to be smashed, and tractor and truck engines need to be started every few hours.

At about four p.m., the phone rang. A former neighbor called from town asking if we could check on the horse she boarded at a farm about a mile and a half down the road from us. Apparently the horse—a colt bred from her Appaloosa mare and Kathi's Tennessee Walking Horse stallion, creating what is known as a Walkaloosa—was down in these subzero temperatures. "Would you take it a blanket?" she asked. It was ten below zero, with winds gusting between thirty and forty miles per hour, meaning the wind chill was minus fifty degrees. A blanket is all it needed?

When Kathi returned from answering that call and rushed through the door, I knew something was terribly, terribly wrong. A trainer for twenty-five years, Kathi was well acquainted with all aspects of equine care, including rescue. Seeing just how scared Kathi was for this animal, I didn't hesitate to grab the truck keys, bundle up in several layers of clothes, and head back outside.

Thoughts of why an animal was out in these conditions and what in the world the farm's owners were doing about it followed me into the cold. Kathi was searching for something to transport the downed horse across the pasture in, while I fired up a very cold diesel truck and started hooking up the horse trailer. Everything takes longer in this cold, but we were on our way in under an hour.

For a second I looked up from hitching the trailer to see what Kathi found to move the horse across the snow: an old orange plastic child's sled we had sitting in the barn. Just how small was he anyway?

I couldn't see the horse yet, but as soon as I opened the truck door, I could hear him, even over the thirty-mile-an-hour winds. The farm boarding this horse sits atop a hill, a ways from the main road, at the end of a long driveway. The winds here were whipping so fast and, as they raced across the open fields, picked up ice, which splintered into flying shards, stinging our eyes. It literally took my breath away out in that openness, and I had to breathe in short rasps to avoid hurting my throat and lungs.

The blowing snow made it even harder to see. Kathi and I had to squint to protect our eyes. As I looked through the snow a dark shape, flat against the ground, was becoming visible. We started to cross the yard, and there he was, lying down in an open field, near the property fence. Even through the howling wind I could hear his high-pitched, scared whinny piercing through the storm. There was no doubt in my mind this horse was calling for help the second he heard the truck doors slam.

As soon as I saw him, I quickly returned to the truck to maneuver it and the trailer through a narrow area between the farm owner's home and their barn, so the trailer would be closer to the horse. As I backed the trailer to the edge of the yard, I noticed the back of the house had a wide dining room window overlooking the area where Kathi and I were headed. It turned out the farm's owners were actually home. We later learned that for six hours, the people boarding this horse, a husband and wife, watched him from this window. The wife, who owned the farm, thought it was "cute"—her words—how he lay there all day. From ten that morning, they watched him and heard his cries.

Kathi and I went to the door to explain to the farm owner why we were here. "Are you finally here to help the little horse?" asked a little boy, no more than four years old, when the door opened after Kathi knocked. At least somebody here cared, I thought. Kathi quickly explained to the farm owners that the downed horse's owner called and asked us to care for him, and that Kathi and I thought it best if we brought him back to our farm for care. There was no argument. In fact, they made it clear they wanted the horse gone, that they had never agreed to provide it shelter, and that this "wasn't their responsibility." The husband came out to help load him, telling us the entire time he didn't want the animal dying on their property.

He also tried to claim the colt had access to food. We knew from experience this was not the case—sometimes smaller, weaker horses will be chased away from food by older, stronger horses. An alert, caring boarding farm owner would realize what was going on and rectify the situation.

It took all of us—Kathi, the farm owner's husband, and me—a few minutes to trudge through the snow and ice the hundred or so yards to where the horse lay. As I got closer, what I saw and heard is forever etched in my mind. The horse was frantically jerking his head, trying to turn toward us, his whinny getting higher with our every step. The sound of a baby horse's whinny is usually one of the most joyful sounds, like a young child laughing and playing. This was a helpless, terrified sound, and it didn't stop until we reached him.

The reason he sounded so frantic, as if he were trapped, was that he was. Lying before me was a very young horse frozen to the ground. Along with his head, he could move part of his neck, and that was it. The warmth of his body had melted a concave impression into the ice, freezing him into place. His back legs had frozen extended straight outward. His front legs were frozen in a fetal position where he had gone down.

Having seen a number of once strong animals decimated by maltreatment, Kathi knew this horse was at an even greater disadvantage, because he was so young—only nine months old. But even an untrained observer looking across the fence at his prone body would have known immediately it was down due to starvation. His skeleton showed through the skin draped loosely over it. His neck was half the thickness it should have been. He was gaunt, weak, and literally just bones. His ribs, hips, and shoulders were clearly visible. The average weight of a nine-month-old colt is around 750 pounds. This little guy weighed maybe half that.

When we got to him, his cry stopped. I couldn't believe this little horse was still alive. He must have had an unbelievable will to live. I looked down at the orange sled Kathi was holding and wondered how this was going to get him across the pasture and through the yard to the trailer. We knelt down and touched him. With the wind pounding the chill deeper into him with each passing second, we looked into his desperate—yet hopeful—eyes. They pleaded with us to please help him. "Please don't go away again," they seemed to say.

Running our hands over his limbs we realized this little being was not merely cold or frostbit or slightly hypothermic. He was frozen solid. The only parts of his body that worked at that point were his head and neck, which was apparent by how he had kept twisting his head toward the house and driveway when he called to us for help.

The three of us lifted him high enough to wedge the sled under his body. The hole his body had made in the ice was about six to eight inches deep. Kathi maneuvered the sled as the men lifted his body. With his body so frozen the best we could do was roll him. His coat was thick with ice. Each time I felt his frozen legs I cringed. There was no flexibility. He was truly frozen. Through it all, the little colt lay there, not moving, not making a sound. He seemed to instinctively know we were trying to help him.

While the farm owner's husband pulled the sled like a mad man across that yard, I pushed and tried to keep his body on the little sled. Throughout the entire time he kept saying, "I don't want this horse to die on our property. I just want him out of here." He was pulling the sled too fast. I repeatedly yelled at him to slow down, because the horse was slipping off. His back legs were extended, so every drift and bump in the snow jarred him off the sled. The man seemed not to care, intent only on getting the horse to that trailer and gone forever.

Once we arrived at the trailer, he started to manhandle the colt into it. This trailer has a divider at the door that cannot be removed. Since the horse's legs couldn't be bent, the guy kept pulling on the halter, all the while continuing his rant. I finally told him to stop pulling and get out. Kathi and I finished loading the horse into the trailer, while the man headed back to the house without a word. We took some solace in the fact that at least the colt couldn't feel any of the pain this guy would have caused him. Under normal circumstances, dragging a prone horse through a door that way could have broken his legs. But there wasn't anything normal about these circumstances.

Relieved to finally be on our way and away from this place, we closed the trailer doors and headed for the truck. Neither of us spoke. What was there to say after that experience? And we both wanted out of there as quickly as possible. I think the little horse felt the same way. He was quiet. Not even a whimper. When we closed the door to the trailer, his only reaction was to watch us.

Finally, this little colt was going home.

2

Warming Back to Life

Turning into our driveway, I slowed the truck, mindful of the frail figure resting behind us. I didn't want the ice ruts to jar the trailer. It was dusk now, and in our winters the sky appears heavier with the coming dark, like the cold is weighing it down. Despite the cold and the dark, almost every time the house first comes into view I recall another afternoon, a much warmer and far greener one, three years earlier.

Raindance Farms opened its gates in 2005, the result of a dream to live in the country and a relatively newfound love of horses. I had always wanted to ride horses, but I'd only begun riding two years prior. When I'd hit my midthirties, I realized it was time to actually do it or quit talking about it and find a new dream. The only previous exposure I had to horses was when I was little and my cousin put me on her Arabian—bareback—and wished me luck. Needless to say, I survived.

So many years later, I asked a friend with horses if she'd take me riding. During that first ride as an adult, I found a home I had been missing all these years. The horse, Tootsie (though I refused to ride a horse named Tootsie, so my friend let me call her Diablo), decided she would test me and took off across a pasture.

Immediately, my friend yelled something, but I couldn't hear it. I think it was something about not damaging her horse. Regardless, we found out that day I was a natural. For whatever reason, God gave me an inherent ability to ride and to react appropriately without thinking when a horse does the unexpected. To this day my friend good-naturedly teases me about being able to ride like that when it takes others years of training.

What started as a simple question of whether or not I could ride quickly became an all-consuming hobby. Now it's a lifestyle. I may never become a professional show rider, but the upside is I don't want to. I went from begging to ride a friend's horse to leasing one to finally owning my first horse. Her barn name was Rain, and I formally registered her as "A Dance in the Rain." Sounded like a good name for a new farm, too.

But I was only halfway there. The remainder of my farm's name came from a horse owned by a woman I met when buying Rain. Searching for my first horse meant weeding through a pile of ads. One of the people I called was Kathi Davis, a lifelong horse person, who was reducing the size of her herd. None of her horses met the needs of a beginner, but she pointed me to the right people. A path that led to Rain.

After learning I purchased Rain, she sent me a congratulatory e-card. Not long after that, a friend, who denies it to this day, volunteered me to chair the public relations committee for the Minnesota Walking Horse Association—a great idea given I had been involved with this breed for less than a year and was still learning to ride. Kathi e-mailed me more congratulations, and I wrote back thanking her, and said that I considered her my first recruit to the committee and welcome aboard.

I soon discovered Kathi owned Dance, who was Rain's mom. Our committee work led to a relationship that led me to look for a larger place in the country than I originally anticipated. Having found the perfect place, I started brainstorming names the very day its previous owners accepted my offer.

The property is located at the top of a hill overlooking Lake Superior and the surrounding countryside. There is almost always a breeze or wind. Standing in its driveway one late summer afternoon in 2005, the farm named itself with a mist rolling in and a gentle rain falling. It dawned on me the mist and rain were swirling, dancing in the wind. It didn't hurt that my first horse, Rain, was standing in the same pasture as her dam, Dance.

Kathi brought her horses and would operate her horse-training business at the same location, so the name needed a plural, thus, "Raindance Farms" was born. When you first achieve a dream, you often spend a lot of time standing next to it and smiling. Even when it's raining. I had wanted a place in the country all my life and here it was.

Three years later, as we drove up to the barn with a frozen horse behind us in the trailer, we were reminded how we pay for those warm, gentle summer rains in these parts six months later when a biting cold can freeze water into crystals before it hits the ground. When we arrived at the house, Kathi called a friend, David, from a neighboring farm and asked if he could help us unload the horse.

While waiting for David to arrive, we ransacked the house, grabbing everything we could find that could create warmth: blankets off beds, space heaters, a blow-dryer. The doorbell rang, but it wasn't our friend. The horse's owner and her boyfriend were at the door. She was, by all appearances, intoxicated. Making matters worse, she was not dressed for this weather, further putting herself at risk. Once assured we would soon find a place for him in the barn, she left saying she had to go feed her kids. We would see her only once more. After

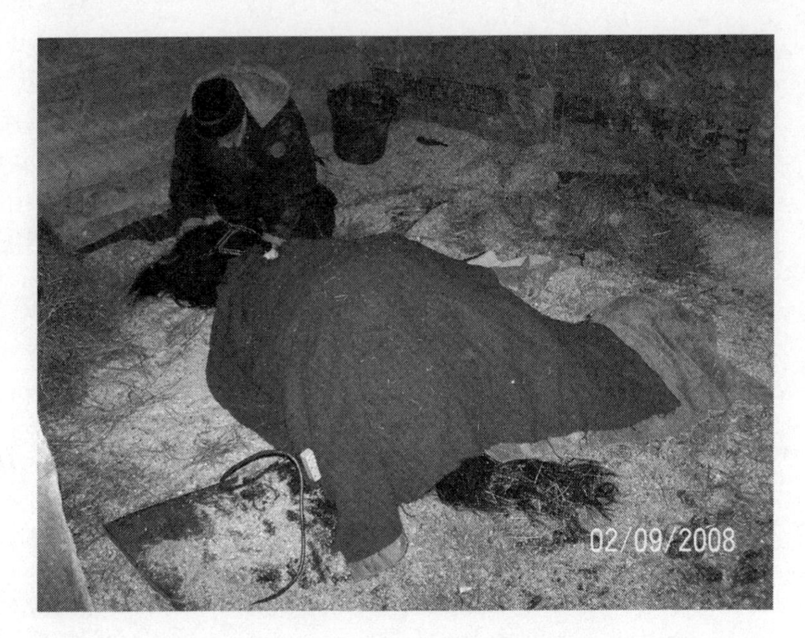

Windchill with volunteer David S. (photo by Jeffrey L. Tucker)

several phone conversations, she eventually transferred ownership of the horse to Kathi.

David arrived about a half hour after they left. Within minutes we had a plan for moving the colt once he was out of the trailer. We slid a tarp under him, and then dragged him across the pen and into stall 5, which we had prepared with some hay, straw, and towels. Due to the extreme conditions, inside the barn it felt nearly indistinguishable from the outside. The heaters made very little headway in such a large open space. So we called the other horses into the barn to allow their body temperature to raise the temperature of the air surrounding the downed horse.

The other horses raced into the barn, headed for their stalls, and braked to a halt when they heard a noise from stall 5. From that point they knew. They knew there was a seriously injured being in there. They looked at one another and whinnied as if asking, "How can we help?" They looked over at him as they quietly munched, and Windchill took notice. All he had known of older, bigger horses was how they basically ignored him or ran him off the hay piles where he was boarded. Now he was probably wondering once again, "How come they can eat and I can't?"

Our barn has six stalls, and we had horses in each one at the time. We chose stall 5 for Windchill's home so he could have horses in the stalls on both sides of him every night. Over the next twenty days, we always had at least one of our three "moms" with him, day and night: Dance, Grace, or Bonnie, or our one grandma, Annie, a twenty-five-year-old crabby old mare with a fondness for youngsters.

After getting all the horses in the barn, we scoured the house for supplies. When we were finished, not a towel or blanket was left in the house. If it was dry, it came outside and became one of the many layers that enfolded the colt. Gently, we began the process of thawing his joints. Using a blow-dryer, it took almost two and a half hours to warm one leg to the point where we could start bending it at the knee.

In a way, it was here in our barn where this little guy was reborn. Before now, the barn's frozen stillness was broken only once in a while by a horse's shudder. But tonight, the quiet was shattered by the constant whine of a blow-dryer. Bringing this tiny colt back. Limb by frozen limb.

3

The First Night

I can't begin to imagine what it felt like for this little horse as his limbs started to thaw. I suffered frostbite myself, and even a touch of hypothermia, when I fell through the ice in the harbor near Lake Superior when I was in high school. Fortunately, my brother was there to pull me out. I can still remember that "pins and needles" sting in my legs as circulation returned. But for the colt, his entire body was frozen. The intense ache that accompanies thawing was going to last several days, not just a few minutes.

One might expect this severely weakened colt to be extremely lethargic after all he had suffered, partly out of exhaustion, partly out of resignation to his current state. But he was conscious and alert the entire time. It was clear to us that much of his body was not working, but his eyes were surprisingly clear. We knew he was aware of his surroundings. Those eyes were clearly observing, curious as to what we were doing. Since he hadn't connected with caregivers in obviously quite some time, I suppose he was wondering why we were doing this, why we were bothering.

I think this curiosity stoked his motivation to keep living from the moment he arrived at our place. He wanted to know what would happen next and why. I think he liked getting to know us, so he lay there quietly, hour after hour, and let us work. Despite what had to be incredible pain, he never complained, never groaned, cried out, or winced. After he was settled in his stall for a while, he finally got to eat. We turned off the blow-dryer, and he quietly munched. And munched and munched. We held him in our laps with a water bucket for him to drink from time to time. And then he'd munch some more.

Every moment of that first night found us astonished he was still alive. How he survived out there in that pasture for hours in those elements is a testament to his willpower, to his desire to live. Why he would want to continue living under those circumstances is anyone's guess. So there we were, out in the dull yellow buzz of the barn lights at night, the wind howling outside the barn and sneaking in from time to time from underneath the big doors and through the rafters. While kneeling next to him, we started to serenade the little colt again with a blow-dryer and tried to imagine what the last twelve hours had been like for him.

If he survived the night, we discussed how he would need a strictly controlled diet, lots of water, and nonstop care in order to, someday, get him back on his feet. If he survived the night. We were skeptical he would. But we continued to try bringing his body temperature up as best we could. We rested him on layers of straw covered by blankets. This created an insulating layer between him and the floor. The blankets protected his paper-thin skin from the straw.

It was Carhartts all around for us, bundled layer upon layer, but the cold still worked its way into our bones. Meanwhile, this tiny horse had been frozen to the ground with high winds and ice shards lashing his eyes and flesh. It stung us the brief while we were out

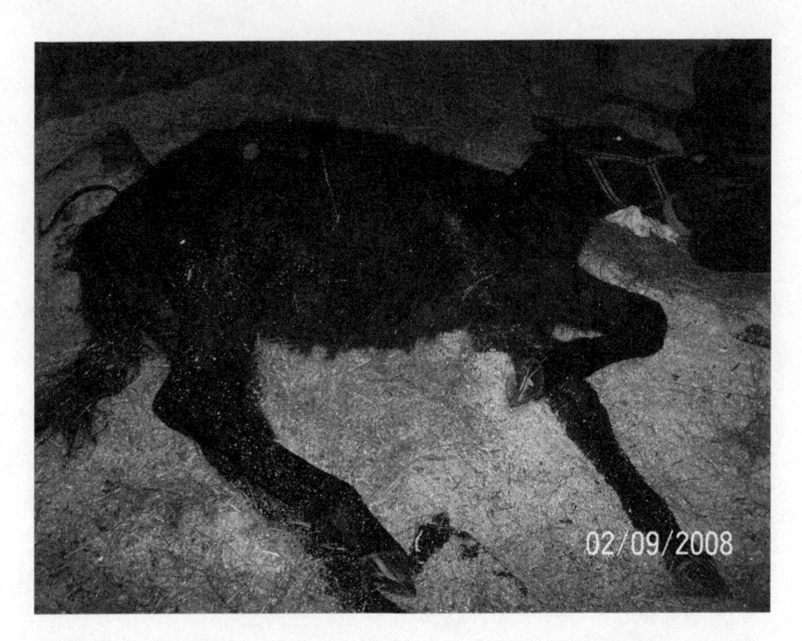

A very thin Windchill immediately after being rescued (photo by Jeffrey L. Tucker)

there, so heaven only knows what it felt like to him. Although there must have been a point when he stopped feeling the cold due to numbness, eventually the numbness melted away here in the barn, exposing him to the pain all over again.

The heaters in the barn did little but take the edge off the cold, but rotating towels constantly helped accelerate the drying process. After blow-drying for more than two hours, the ice melted out of his coat, and he was dry to the touch. The night wore on with rotations of lifting him up to water and keeping hay at the ready for munching. Most helpful that first night was the constant company of the other horses. We later reflected that his having this company was likely one of the most important things that kept him going that night, along with his faith in us.

Knowing we had a clear case of neglect lying here in our barn, we took photos of his frail body. Unfortunately we started taking pictures after we dried him, so his coat was much fuller and it partially hid his emaciated shape. Kathi's extensive experience with rescue horses had not prepared even her for what we documented. In a way, he was a "perfect storm" of neglect: dehydrated, malnourished, and suffering from hypothermia and possible frostbite. Two vets who visited him as well as others we consulted would later confirm it was if not the worst case of starvation and neglect they had ever seen then near the top of the list.

No longer content with just calling our new friend "him" or "little guy," we decided on a name. His original name was Diamond, likely due to the marking on his forehead. However, he rarely saw his original owner, and knowing the lack of care he'd had up until tonight, we doubted he even knew his name, because no one ever told him.

So once the blow-dryer was turned off for the night, and we were just sitting with him, holding him up for another drink, Kathi said, "We should call him Windchill." I nodded and smiled, since it fit perfectly. Even he seemed to like it.

Despite surviving all that time in the pasture and now quietly enduring the pain of thawing out, Windchill's eyes never lost their searching interest in us and his new home. They also never lost their glow. It was like a flickering candle. It might dim for a second, but always brightened again. We hoped and prayed that that flicker, along with his need to know what would happen next, was enough to carry him through to morning.

We stayed with him until about 2:30 a.m. There was nothing more we could do, so we went inside. We knew we were doing all we could. The rest was in his and God's hands.

About four hours after leaving the barn, we returned, slightly rested, not sure what awaited us behind its doors. What we found

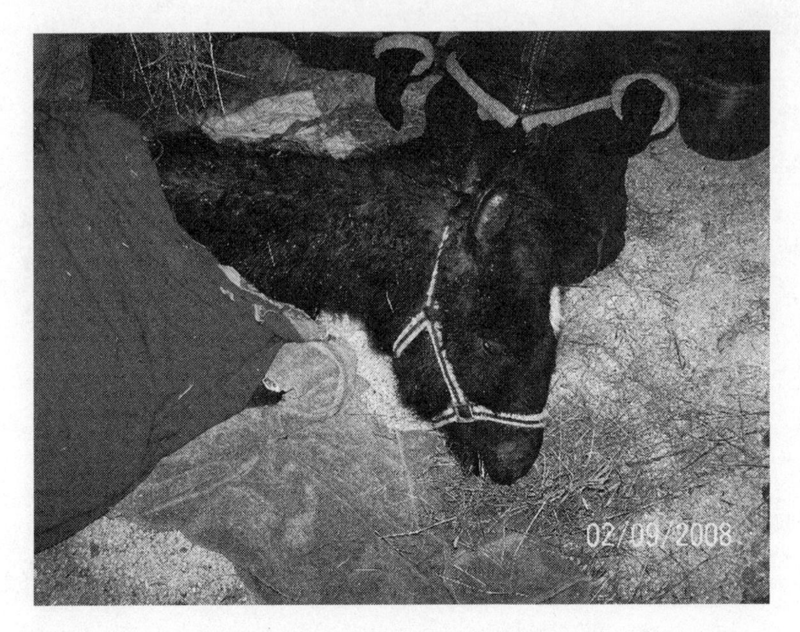

Windchill munches on hay the night of the rescue (photo by Jeffrey L. Tucker)

was a little colt not only alive, but whinnying a welcome as we entered. This whinny sounded less frightened than what we first heard in yesterday's driving wind. But I could hear a hint of worry, like he knew he still had a long road back. Despite all he had been through, he was in no way lethargic. His eyes were alert, and he stretched his neck gingerly to look around as much as he could. The message to us was clear: Windchill made a choice that night, a choice to live.

So we made up our minds as well to help him do just that. We never looked back after that morning. We propped up his body with hay bales, so he could view his surroundings more comfortably and continue to munch. Despite the pain, discomfort, and determined hold the cold had on him he had such a sweet, cheerful personality. Our vet would later say that Windchill, a Tennessee Walking Horse

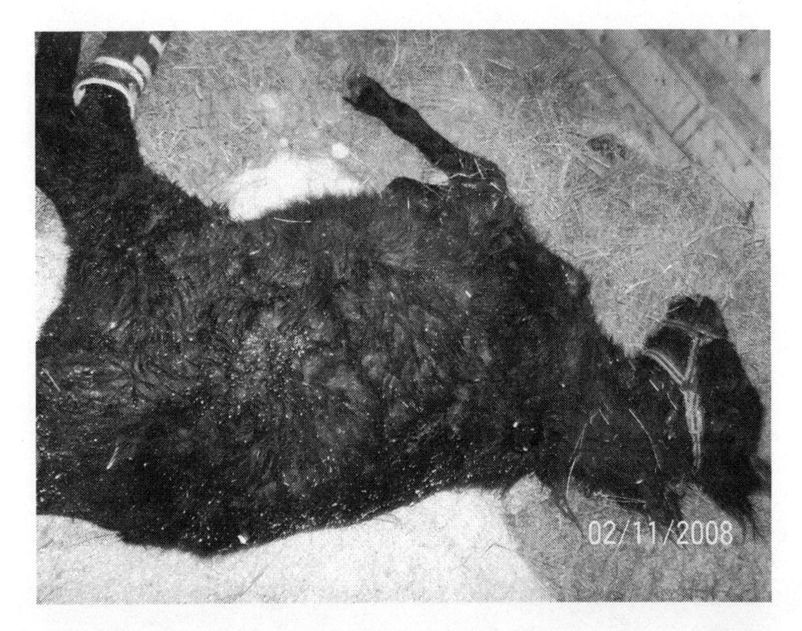

Now that his hair is dry it masks the frail and thin colt's body (photo by Jeffrey L. Tucker)

and Appaloosa cross, probably got his sweet temperament from the Walker side, and his stubborn refusal to do anything but live from the Appaloosa side. Imagine a person out there in the cold and wind for hours, starving. Grateful for the rescue, yes, but cheerful? I doubt it.

David and another friend, Stacy, visited that morning. Their attachment to Windchill was almost as immediate as ours. They would soon join us as the founding members of "Team Windchill." Little did any of us know that Sunday how many sleepless nights, cups of coffee, and hours consulting with equine experts and authorities awaited us in the very near future.

The first veterinarian to visit was our own farm vet who came that Sunday. Her orders to us were to keep him hydrated, warm, and

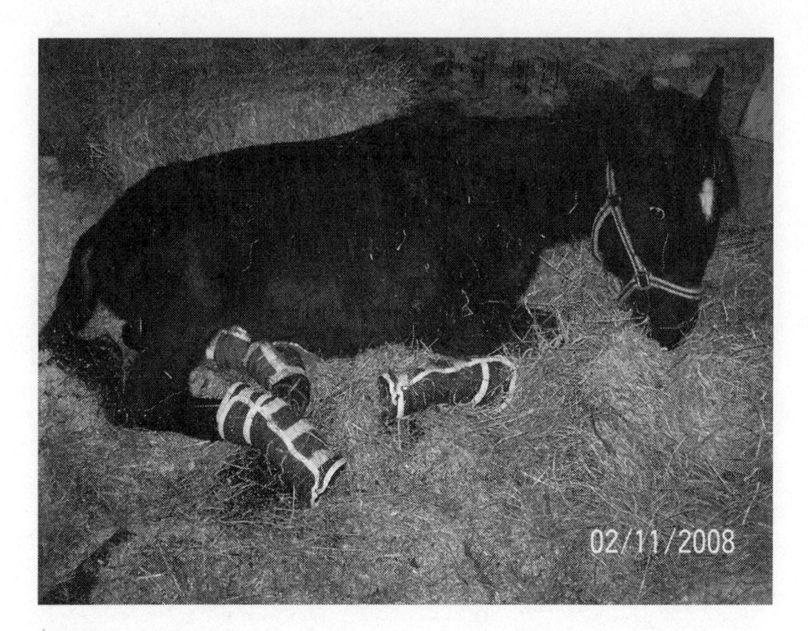

Windchill lies resting on straw with socks to warm his legs (photo by Jeffrey L. Tucker)

dry. Another vet would later suggest we might need to put him down. That vet couldn't pick up a pulse in his legs. But this diagnosis didn't add up with the slight warmth we were starting to detect in the legs and Windchill's attempts to move them. This was the first of many dismissals of Windchill's chances, but he had survived that first night. We felt we owed him a fighting chance.

That and seeing his eyes shine brighter than ever that morning told us he was more than ready to fight.

4

Team Windchill Goes Worldwide

At first, it was just David, Stacy, Kathi, and me. By Monday, our friends the Bresnahan family were regulars on the Windchill watch. Over the next nineteen days, Windchill's stall became a second home to these people. This amazing, seemingly tireless core group put much of their regular lives on hold and scraped every possible spare minute for time at Raindance. Their presence made it possible for Kathi and me to sneak in a power nap, a meal, or online time with equine experts.

The Internet fast became another, powerful member of our team. At first, Kathi and I just scouted advice from experts regarding how to treat Windchill. In a matter of days, though, this modern, instantaneous connection to the world became a lifeline. Not only did our research about how to care for Windchill start here, but whenever we needed assistance, people replied almost immediately.

For example, the University of California–Davis website and forums were a wealth of information for us. A contact there messaged

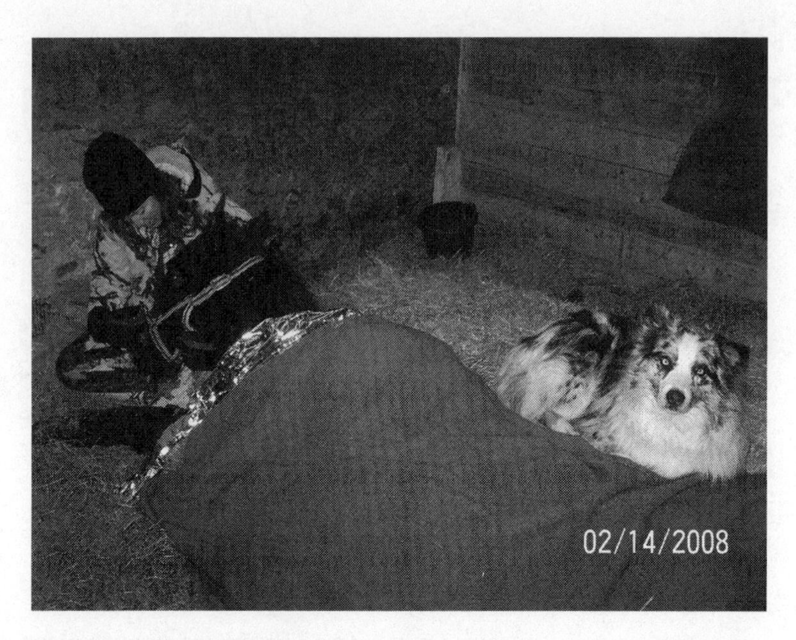

A volunteer, Kris B., stands watch over Windchill along with our dog, Walker (photo by Jeffrey L. Tucker)

us that Windchill's diet needed to incorporate more alfalfa. Finding alfalfa locally was next to impossible. When I mentioned our alfalfa problem online, a woman from northeastern Wisconsin named Vicki Knutson answered within eight minutes. She drove alfalfa squares to us within a day, about two hours each way, and wouldn't take any money.

Windchill's days of anonymity were soon past. State law requires that, in the case of possible animal maltreatment, a court-appointed vet must examine the animal. On Tuesday, the sheriff finally found a vet who could be at our farm that afternoon. We suspected the diagnosis would be the path of least resistance, meaning we'd be told to put the horse down. So I called the local newspaper, the *Duluth News Tribune*, asking if they would be interested in the story of a nine-month-old colt who had been left to freeze in a pasture, and a number of people were doing all they could to save him, and you should just see the spirit this little guy is showing, and the sheriff was coming with a vet to tell us we might have to put him down . . . They had a photographer and reporter to the farm by the time the sheriff and vet had arrived.

The sheriff's vet did recommend putting Windchill down, but the newspaper ran the story the next day, front page. As a result people started coming to Raindance in droves. Some called ahead, some didn't, but many of them offered to help. By now, we were in the barn almost all the time. All of us still had farms to operate and full-time off-farm jobs. The hours were adding up fast, and each of us was starting to use paid time off. Our nights were quickly eaten up by the things we didn't get done during the day, so many of these offers to help were accepted readily.

Some of our first volunteers were people who lived in the area, stopped in to see Windchill, and realized how thinly stretched we were. This is one way the Windchill family grew. These folks told their friends about Windchill, and soon, more people would be offering to help.

Another way the family grew was thanks to that first newspaper story. The story spread like wildfire across the Internet, getting posted on blogs around the country. Shortly after it was printed, one of our volunteers told me she had Googled "Windchill" and our names. She found nearly twenty-five thousand websites had posted the article.

People wanting updates on Windchill's recovery started overwhelming the *Duluth News Tribune* and the sheriff's office with calls the very day the article ran. The paper wanted to create a blog for me on their website, because they were unable to handle the volume of calls. But since I already had the Raindance website, I figured it would be easier to link to a blog there, and have the paper and sheriff's office give people our web address for updates about Windchill. Thus, the Windchill blog began that day.

Once the *Duluth News Tribune* story ran, other media outlets started calling. Television and radio stations from Duluth and the Twin Cities not only picked up the story but also followed up with regular updates. I learned a morning host with Minnesota Public Radio was updating listeners each morning by checking my blog. A reporter from KARE-11 in Minneapolis sent a reporter here for the day. A reporter from a local station, WDIO-TV, not only covered the story but later brought his family out to see Windchill.

The blog began getting hits from all over the country right away, and within a couple days, from all over the world. People told me my posts were getting reposted all over the Internet. Discussion groups about Windchill were forming on many other sites. No matter how tired I was or how little time there was to spare, I wanted to keep people informed. It was like I owed it to them. The quantity and depth of concern was that great.

So many people took the time to comment, not just once but often on a daily basis. Their cheers, prayers, and continuous encouragements reminded us—as if we needed reminding—that Windchill was truly special. Just like all of us caring for Windchill at Raindance, these people wanted him to survive, to beat the odds—to show the folks who wrote him off that they were wrong.

A few celebrities even chimed in. A member of the Windchill forum faithful e-mailed me, "Hey, you guys just got a shout out from the Allman Brothers!"

> Dear Windchill and your wonderful care providers, on behalf of the Allman Brothers Band and its extended family, collectively known as the Peach Corps, "Go Windchill, go!" We're zenning endless positive, healing vibes your way and pray for your complete recovery. Take care and know that you are loved.

Here are just a few of the messages we received on the Windchill forum. These messages echo what thousands of others were also posting.

Sandy H: Hang in there Windchill, you are getting the best care from the best people there is. My donation will be in the mail soon. Thank you to all of you that are spending your time caring for Windchill, he is so cute on TV and to see him pawing at the hay is so hard to believe!! Keep it up!

The Radtkes: We are so excited to learn that Windchill is making such wonderful progress. I've shared the story with my 5- and 7-year-old children which has really touched us all. They asked about him right away this morning when they woke up and I will be so happy to report the good news back to them. I commend you for taking the initiative and responsibility to help in this situation when his owner did not. Your act of kindness has prompted others to get involved . . . [I]t seems the "pay it forward" mentality is in full swing. The first thing I do each morning is check your website for an update and I appreciate you taking the time to do this knowing full well you are probably exhausted. While our family has no experience working with horses (just our beloved dog!), we are animal lovers. I'm sure you have had many visitors and if visiting is still an option, I know my kids would love to take a peek at the horse that has captured the hearts of many. Thank you for all you have done and continue to do!

Denis and Susan in Arizona: Dear little Windchill—We are on your site more than several times a day checking on you—we are so worried for your welfare and are praying constantly for you and your AWESOME caregivers. We wish so much that we lived close by so we could help everyone out—even doing chores for Jeff and

Kathi so they can spend more time with you, or bringing food for everyone and fresh blankets. Since distance prevents that, all we can do is keep sending you donations, which we will continue to keep doing as long as it takes to get you completely healed. Take care little one. Much love.

Lynette H: Our prayers are with you—may you continue to heal—God has truly touched you and given you LOTS of guardian angels!!

Greg T: I'm not a horse owner, but my heart goes out to this little guy. You folks who are helping this colt are a fantastic example of what a Human Being really is! How can this effort fail with all the good that is in that barn everyday!

Diane M: Sweet little guys like Windchill are so easy to rally for. Caring for the innocent and vulnerable seems to bring out the tenderness in all of us. I believe daily we need to love each other with the same amount of compassion and passion that has been shown to Windchill. God Bless, Diane

Bill and Tracey: We have followed this story since day 1 and are so excited to see that Windchill is doing so well! As animal lovers of all kinds seeing any pet in pain just breaks our hearts. Hugs to Windchill and hats off to all who have worked to save him!

Amy T: Windchill you are a "Miracle." I am so amazed at how far you have come. Your caregivers sound like amazing people who never stopped fighting for you . . . [T]hey are truly god's hand and heart. They have given you strength to fight and love to survive. You will always be one of a kind. God bless all of you caregivers.

Darlene B in Hawaii: I wish you all strength & serenity during these difficult times. My heart hurts for Windchill. My husband and myself check your website many times daily. My husband comes home from work and asks 'how's the little guy today?' I wish I could help.

Kathy T: Read the update on Windchill this morning once I got to the office, and did some crying. I'm sure everyone wants what is best for Windchill. It's all about Windchill's comfort, health, and quality of life. You all are the horse experts, and also have vets and healers there to give you their advice about what is best for Windchill now. With all of the compassion, wisdom, and competence that you all have shown thus far, I am confident that whatever decision you all make will be in the best interest of Windchill. Sunflower thoughts and heartfelt prayers keep being sent to all from Kathy, Cisco and Jazz (the Tonk furballs) in Kansas.

Mary Jane in Indiana: Good evening Little Fellow. I wish you sweet dreams tonight. May your indomitable spirit sustain and nourish you. You have many of us pulling for you.

Jennifer: What a great story. There is hope for us all.

I think this last comment does the best job of explaining why so many people cared.

Windchill's national following grew dramatically when Fox News called and said Jane Skinner wanted to do a story on her morning news show about us. I asked, "Jane who?" and they were shocked to learn I had not watched television since 1996, the very same year Fox debuted in a few markets. Due to scheduling conflicts, there was no way to conduct an in-studio interview, so I sent them as many pictures and videos as I could and Jane interviewed me over the phone. The results were immediate.

I was at my desk at work when the interview took place, and happened to glance at my computer monitor and e-mail display while talking with Jane. The e-mail counter starting ticking upward quickly. The interview was not even finished and my inbox was bursting. I thought my spam filter must have shut down. I hung up and found out quickly that Fox News is apparently aired EVERYWHERE now. I opened my e-mail box and messages were pouring in from all over the country. On a whim, I thought I had better check the blog. It was moving very, very slowly. And then it crashed. All within seven minutes of the interview.

After it crashed, I called the company that hosted our site, asked if they were having problems, and a resounding, slightly annoyed "Yes!" was the reply. Turns out their server had to be rebooted due to a flood of viewers. While I explained what was going on, I looked up the bandwidth meter for our website. This meter never meant anything to me before, because we never came close to meeting our monthly limit. But now the meter was soaring. I told them I couldn't afford this if it kept climbing. They told me not to worry about it. They would open up the bandwidth and take care of the cost. Our first corporate donation.

Our site's typical daily number of hits would be in the low hundreds at most. After the *Duluth News Tribune* story, it climbed significantly. Within a week of getting reposted across the World Wide Web, 750,000 to 1 million viewers were reading about Windchill on our site. After the Fox story, we peaked at about 3.5 million. It would eventually average to approximately 100,000 views a day for the duration of Windchill's time with us.

Shortly after announcing on the blog that we built a guest registry where people could comment, we tried printing the comments out—good reading material for our shifts in the barn. We stopped printing them out after four hours, because it was consuming too much paper. But we taped twelve pages of them up in Windchill's stall to cheer him up.

Two days later a volunteer managed to print the entire log up to that point in time. It filled a thick three-ring binder, and we kept that in his stall, too. This attention was uplifting, energizing and draining all at once. The phone literally never quit ringing. No sooner did we empty the answering machine of messages, and it was full again. Most were well-wishers, with lots of advice. Some of it was funny, but I couldn't laugh. They were so sincere. People were calling with advice from their experience with dogs, cats, hamsters, and guinea pigs. Advice that may not translate too well to horse care. Someone swore on a stack of saddles giving Windchill large doses of cayenne pepper was the answer.

People were telling me they were so riveted to the blog updates, they had to discipline themselves or risk getting behind at work. One woman, an attorney from Texas, took the time to write me a two-page letter about how moved she was by Windchill's story. She would reward herself if she completed a specific task—such as completing a brief—by allowing herself to check the blog for the latest on Windchill's condition. It was the only way she could get anything done, she said.

The online following was so intense that many readers knew my schedule almost as well as I did. One message on our machine said, "I know from reading your blog that you're already out in the barn by 4:30 a.m., so I knew I could reach you if I called after midnight or before 4 a.m. . . ." People started coming to the farm in such numbers, some even letting themselves into the barn, that we had to ramp up our time staying in the barn with Windchill. On average, fifteen to twenty people would be at the farm at a time.

His days as a lonely, neglected colt were definitely done.

5

Finding the Fight

It was the Wednesday after we found him, the same day the story hit the front page. His front legs were starting to show a bit of flexion for the first time. Windchill was trying to stand. He was getting his legs underneath him and pushing. If he could gather the strength to stand there would be hope. His attempt that day was real progress and just another sign that he was a fighter.

Windchill found all the attention to his liking. Whenever he heard a new voice in the barn, he called out. He loved to lay his head in a willing lap and have his head scratched. If we made the mistake of tending to other chores, he called to us as if to say, "Hey, remember me? I could use a little company, people." He was even endearing when munching his grain. Just like a little kid with an ice-cream cone, he was focused. Maybe he'd steal a quick glance up at us once in a while, but for the most part, it was all about mealtime.

The phone's ring became a constant in our lives. We would leave the house to go check on Windchill, and the ring followed us out the door, right after we just finished a call. It also greeted us when we returned to the house, every time. While Windchill loved all this attention, he found it hard to talk on the cordless in a cold barn.

The variety of things that arrived daily never ceased to amaze us. Sox for Horses, Inc. of Havana, Florida, sent Windchill a box full of "Whinny Warmers"—pull-up socks for horses suffering from circulation problems, especially those that are exacerbated by cold weather. The company, which often donates to horse rescues, wrote on the envelope: "Dear Post Office, Hurry! This horse needs help!" And hurry they did. Although our mail had already arrived that Saturday, the U.S. Postal Service carrier returned in the evening to deliver this package, so we wouldn't have to wait until Monday. I couldn't believe it.

A young man, Jake, who heard of Windchill on the Fans of Barbaro forum, followed Windchill's progress faithfully. Barbaro was an American Thoroughbred who had won the Kentucky Derby in 2006 but shattered his leg two weeks later during the Preakness Stakes, ending his career. After a brave fight involving multiple surgeries, his condition began to deteriorate and he had to be euthanized in January 2007. Jake was very emotional about the abuse Windchill endured. A classical music fan, he burned a CD to play in Windchill's stall, after asking for help on the Barbaro forum. "Does anyone here know what kind of music horses prefer?" he asked there. "I've read that research shows music has healing power."

Jake wrote us, "All too often when words fail, when we think there's nothing even close to saying what we feel, we find someone has already said it with a piece of music. One of the pieces that reminds me the most of Windchill is, oddly enough, 'Moonlight Sonata.' It is one of the most peaceful works I can think of, and it reminds me of that night when a certain creature we all know and love found peace as well."

Folks from the Barbaro forum collected money, so Kennett Florist (Barbaro's florist in Pennsylvania) could send flowers here, as well as send prepared frozen meals here for Kathi and myself.

Countless people were offering support, prayers, supplies and donations to help cover costs. A local feed and supply store gave

Windchill a beautiful black halter. We never expected this outpouring. Racing through life, it's easy to never consider how the strangers we pass by every day might be there for us when we need them. They were also calling the Douglas County sheriff's office, district attorney, and the *Duluth News Tribune*, not only wanting to help but also wanting justice.

Justice never exactly happened. The woman who owned the farm pleaded no contest to one misdemeanor count of failing to provide proper shelter. She was sentenced to forty-five days in jail with release granted for work and child care. She also had to pay a five-hundred-dollar fine and allow law enforcement inspections of her property to check on animals in her care for five years.

Her husband pleaded no contest to one count of failure to provide proper food and water to the colt. He was ordered to pay a two-hundred-dollar fine and agreed to allow law enforcement to inspect his property and any animals he possessed for the next three years as part of a deferred judgment of conviction agreement. If he followed the agreement, the charge would be dismissed, and it was.

None of this, in our opinion, qualifies as "justice." In the coming months, many of us who cared for Windchill would meet again to draft Windchill's Law. We wanted Wisconsin to stiffen fines and penalties for animal abuse cases such as this. We wanted to put an end to a slap on the wrist for sending a helpless creature out to die.

Every morning during the rescue, Kathi rotated the "moms" who watched over Windchill. Annie, a great big, black Tennessee Walking Horse, would receive a well-deserved respite, and Dance, another Tennessee Walker, would saunter in, immediately looking over the stall wall with kind, caring eyes. If any of our mares could have legally adopted Windchill, Dance would have stomped, I mean, signed the papers in a second. Ever since we laid Windchill down in the stall that first Saturday night, Dance doted on him like a mother hen.

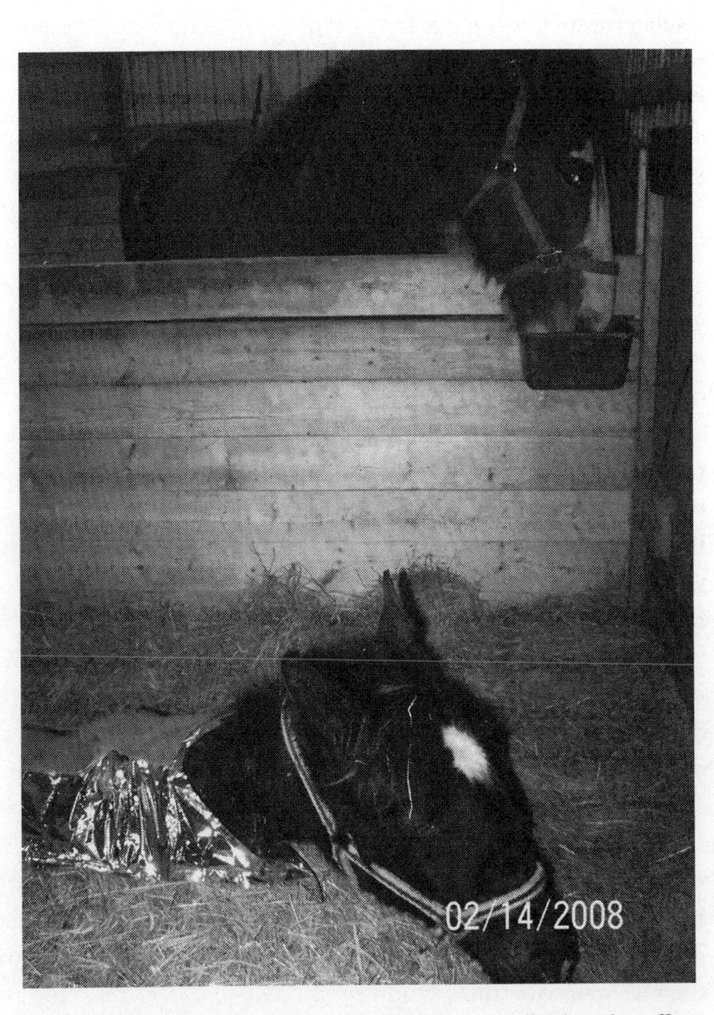

Dance watches over Windchill from the neighboring stall (photo by Jeffrey L. Tucker)

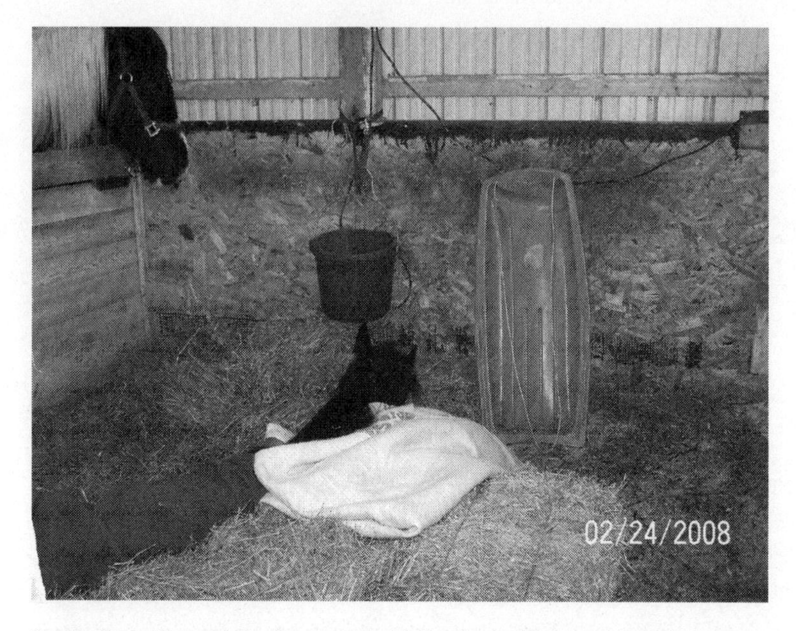

Doting "mom" Bonnie looks over Windchill in his stall; the orange sled is the one used to pull him from the pasture (photo by Jeffrey L. Tucker)

As mother to our farm's namesake, Dance was one of my favorites. Children who visited Raindance loved her and she knew it. Dance had figured out that lowering her head and twisting it just slightly as little ones approached invited a hello pat and, very likely, return visits with treats. She was the most mothering of all Windchill's barn moms. She knew Windchill was terribly fragile, so she hovered about his stall nickering nonstop some days. Windchill appeared most attached to Dance. He started "talking" more when he saw Dance. His ears perked up and his eyes grew wider.

Bonnie and Grace were two of Windchill's other moms. Actually, Grace was more of a great aunt, meaning she was a bit more gruff. Her approach to Windchill was tough love. Grace would grunt at him as if to say, "Oh, just get up already."

Speaking of grace, Bonnie had little. She's a bulldozer of a horse. If Dance was more of a Bloomingdales shopper, Bonnie was all Walmart. A new mare on our farm, she had been owned by cowboys before coming here. Windchill and Bonnie became fast friends. Bonnie was immediately drawn to him, watching him closely, lowering her head over the stall, and nickering to him. Later, Bonnie would be purchased by a Windchill fan in Canada named Darlene who fell in love with the big caring mom and now posts regular pictures of Bonnie's adventures on Facebook.

Now Annie is more of a grandma—not just to Windchill but to all the barn residents. With Windchill, Annie assumed more of a protective guardian role, sizing up each new visitor, then hovering in case they did something she didn't like.

Many of today's Tennessee Walkers seem to be bred more for a smaller, sleeker appearance rather than the large powerhouses of the past bred for crossing the big plantations. Annie was part of an original bloodline. This breed was originally bred to walk great distances across Southern plantations, over rough terrain. Annie was like a big dinosaur, a crabby old mare who towered over the others. One night after lights-out in the barn, I lingered, wondering what these ladies did once the humans left. Annie would take charge is what. She would take center stage in the middle of the aisle and hustle the rest into their stalls. If another horse even so much as turned her head around, Annie pinned her ears back as if to command, "Get back in there!" A warden keeping watch. I left knowing the barn was in good hands.

But Annie's demeanor would completely change once a child was nearby. Like Dance, she'd put her head down in welcome. This explained to us why all of the barn moms, no matter what their personality, were so taken with Windchill. He was a child, and a very sick one at that. He brought out the mother in everyone.

In addition to the horse moms, all of our animals seemed to understand the need to focus their energy on Windchill. Walker, an Australian shepherd, became one of Windchill's best friends. Not only did he sleep with Windchill at night, right next to the colt in his stall, but he deigned to share his precious toys—balls, bones, and the like. Walker never shares. Olivia, the barn cat, slept on him, her body warming his. The moms nickered to him throughout the day.

So with Dance encouraging him, Annie protecting him, the rest of the barn cheering him on, and volunteers helping him get up today, it was safe to predict that he would "stand" an excellent chance of getting to see what the barn looked like beyond the stall.

One morning, when I first went into the barn, there was no movement at all from Windchill. It scared me. I realized at that moment what I wanted for him. I wanted him to live. Before this, during the first three days of Windchill fighting for his life, I wondered what outcome for him would be the best. "If his legs are 'dead,' he has no chance," I thought to myself, "but . . . was that a twitch? Yes, he can move his back legs! Now just move a front one, please . . ."

The ups and downs of caring for a neglected, hurting, and severely malnourished colt are exhausting emotionally and physically. But for that brief moment that morning when I feared he was dead I realized how much I wanted him to live. By the sheer determination he showed trying to stand, I started to believe like never before—maybe, for the first time since we got him—that he would live. And by doing so, he would stand up to the stupidity and downright cruelty of a certain few.

His few attempts to stand that morning wiped him out. One moment he was able to get himself up into a position that allowed him to eat and drink water on his own. Other times he needed help, meaning we had to sit behind him and let him lean on us, or place a wall of hay bales behind him to prop him up.

The Windchill shifts were nearing 24/7. It didn't help the volunteers that the adrenaline rush of the first few days was wearing off and the severe cold was sapping the last of our energy. No matter how many layers, the cold still found its way into joints and muscles. All the volunteers sported dark circles under their eyes. We avoided mirrors altogether. And this was just from sitting with him a couple hours per shift, but almost everyone was coming straight to Raindance from their full-time jobs. Thankfully, some of the phone calls were developing into more volunteers, so the wear and tear eased for a while.

What energized us most was Windchill's drive. After sleeping in another morning, he started flexing his legs and trying to stand again. I wouldn't blame him for stopping after one or two attempts, but he tried standing five times. He refused to give up, which means none of us would either. He was eating and drinking steadily, but we did have to turn him every few hours to avoid stall sores. He was not at all fond of these turns. He would sort of grunt in annoyance. I could understand it: there he was munching away enjoying watching his buddies Dance or Bonnie or Walker, and suddenly someone would block his view and move him out of sight altogether. But the turns had to be done. It took at least two people to turn him and drag him to another part of his stall, where fresh sawdust, clean blankets and hay awaited him.

I stole some time to write on the Windchill blog one morning about how hard he was trying to stand. By that evening, we got a call from a member of the Superior Senior High School faculty. Not only did she offer to join the volunteers of Windchill's care team but her husband offered to develop a lift for us that would utilize our barn rafters. Polly and Gary Niemi would become part of the core Windchill care team, with Gary becoming our official "barn engineer" and Polly sewing up batches of socks for Windchill's legs. It appeared to be the answer to our prayers for a way to get Windchill on his feet. And who knows? Maybe Windchill could get some schooling during his downtime, and the threat of a test would motivate him to stand.

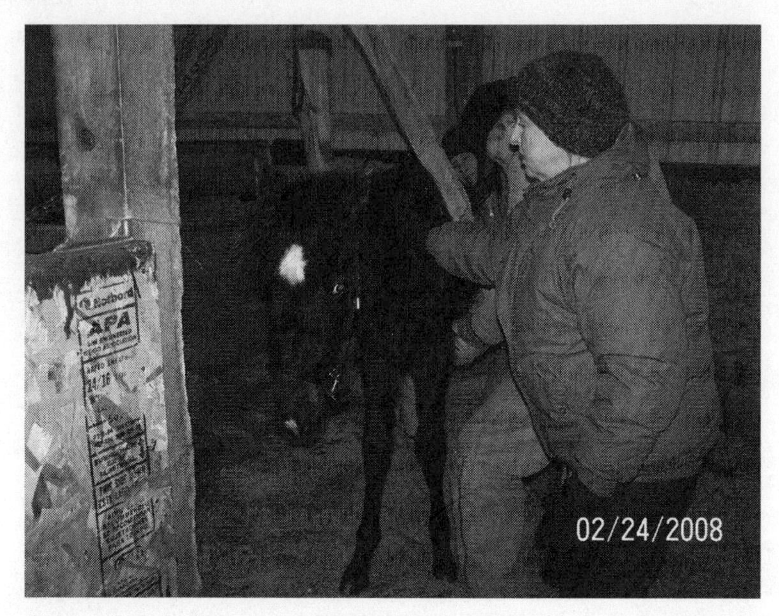

Along with Kathi, barn engineer Gary Niemi and Windchill sock seamstress Polly Niemi ensure none of the materials are rubbing Windchill's thin skin after lifting him to his feet (photo by Jeffrey L. Tucker)

At eleven p.m. on the day he first flexed his front legs, I was in the barn to check on Windchill and give him a final drink. That's when my shift ended and Kathi's would follow. Although he was sleeping much of the day at this point, these attempts to stand drained him completely. I knew he would sleep soundly until the four a.m. shift started. If he was awake at that time, he would be fed, watered, and given meds and fresh blankets.

By Friday, February 15, we saw a significant downturn. Windchill slipped into a serious depression. His whinny that welcomed each turn of the barn door was gone. Head down on a hay bale, his eyes seemed to stare at nothing. I was fearful his spirit was slipping after the failed attempts to stand up. He seemed to be giving up. We were thinking we'd better have him up in the next twenty-four hours, or he'd give up altogether.

My guess was the little guy was frustrated that although his front legs showed more flexibility, his weakness and lack of control overwhelmed his attempts to stand. Compounding the disappointment of the day, an offer of a sling from a local equine association for use with the lift was withdrawn. All we were told was that they didn't feel it would work. We spent the rest of the day racing to find another solution.

One contact lead to another and thankfully, Cindy Aho, of Cloquet, Minnesota, donated the use of her farm's sling and a block-and-tackle winch they used to lift horses and other livestock. If we could muster together enough people, we might be able to lift him the next day.

By late evening, Windchill proved he was a horse of many moods. He went from decidedly depressed, moving very little, and not wanting to sit up at all to perking up as friends came to spend time with him. He even tried to push himself farther up against the hay bales.

The following day was a big one. The vet was coming in the morning. The newspaper was also coming for a follow-up. If the vet gave us the green light, we could try to lift him onto his legs later in the day. If he was to survive, he had to stand. His spirits were worrying us, but that night, after more company, he seemed willing to try and stand again. I was hopeful a week's worth of grain, hay, meds, new friends, and lots of prayer would infuse him with enough drive, energy, and strength to stand all on his own soon.

6

Rising to the Occasion

Late Friday night Windchill slipped back into his funk. Perhaps it was just exhaustion from his earlier efforts to push up on the hay bale. I thought once we started getting him on his feet, his adrenaline would kick in, and he'd want to help.

There would be no lift, though, if our vet found Windchill wasn't ready. After a head-to-hoof exam Saturday, our vet found that although his front legs still lacked a strong pulse, they were warm and he was definitely flexing them. She reassured us by saying the chance Windchill might recover fully was improving. We waited with fingers crossed while she issued a long list of care instructions. Finally, we got the green light to go ahead and lift him onto his legs.

Motivated more than ever, we called the crew that volunteered to help with a lift. Most of the lift crew were members of the Douglas County Sheriff's Department. Many of these folks had visited Windchill throughout the week on their days off. Our other volunteers were neighbors Larry and Char, Gary and Polly Niemi from Superior Senior High, the Dalbec and Bresnahan families, and David.

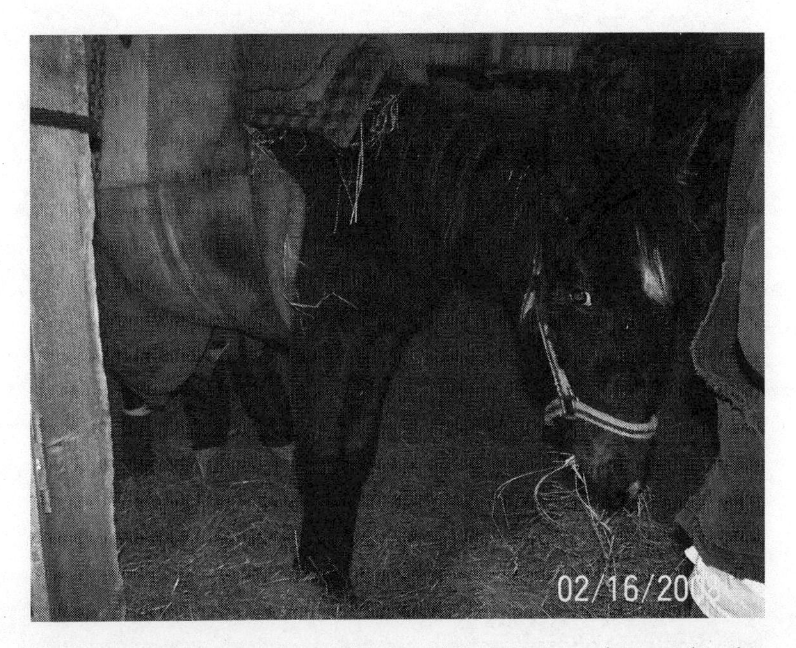

Windchill stands, aided by a blanket-covered hoist to protect his very thin skin (photo by Jeffrey L. Tucker)

Once everyone arrived, we started positioning the sling under Windchill. After he was rolled onto the sling and positioned, the winch was connected to it. Windchill was absolutely calm. He seemed to understand what we were doing. It was as if he knew we needed him to stay calm in order for us to lift him. Hopefully, someday, he could lift his head and neck again and roll onto his sternum by himself, but that was a long time coming, according to the vet. That's okay. We were there to help him.

It was time to start the lift. Everyone not working the winch surrounded Windchill to keep him from sliding out of the sling and to assist with getting his legs under him. The going was rough at first. It was difficult to get his feet in place. But his "landing gear" hit the floor as soon as the sling rose to our knee level. At that point, Windchill did not need the sling anymore.

It was less than two hours since our vet's departure, and we had Windchill standing tall! For the first time since going down in that pasture the previous Saturday, he was up on all fours again. Windchill was on his feet for a full ten minutes.

About three hours later, the same group gathered again to raise Windchill back to his feet. As soon as Windchill heard our voices and the chains of the winch working, he knew what was going down. He let us know he was ready—he prepared by pushing himself off the bales where he was propped up. We found him lying perfectly still, as if he was sleeping with eyes wide open, just waiting.

The second time he stood for twenty minutes! For once, he was less interested in eating and more interested in trying to move. For an animal that has spent the last week thawing out and in many ways coming back to life, these lifts were major workouts. At the end of this lift, he let us know he'd had all he could take by slumping in the sling and going to sleep. We lowered him back to the ground, and he was just able to reposition his legs before drifting off completely.

We had to be very careful of his delicate skin when lifting him in the sling. Within the sling we placed blankets to protect his skin, which could easily tear. For being on his sides so long, he had surprisingly few sores. When standing, we treated the sores with ointment.

It's difficult to describe what it was like seeing him stand there, his eyes bright and excited. He was looking at the world as a horse should: on four legs, standing proud, ready to run, walk, or get into mischief as the other babies on this farm did. I felt like a proud dad. I was also humbled. Windchill's story was spreading across this country like wildfire. The calls continued to come in from all over. Windchill was getting e-mail. I had so underestimated the depth of caring people, what complete strangers are capable of. When we

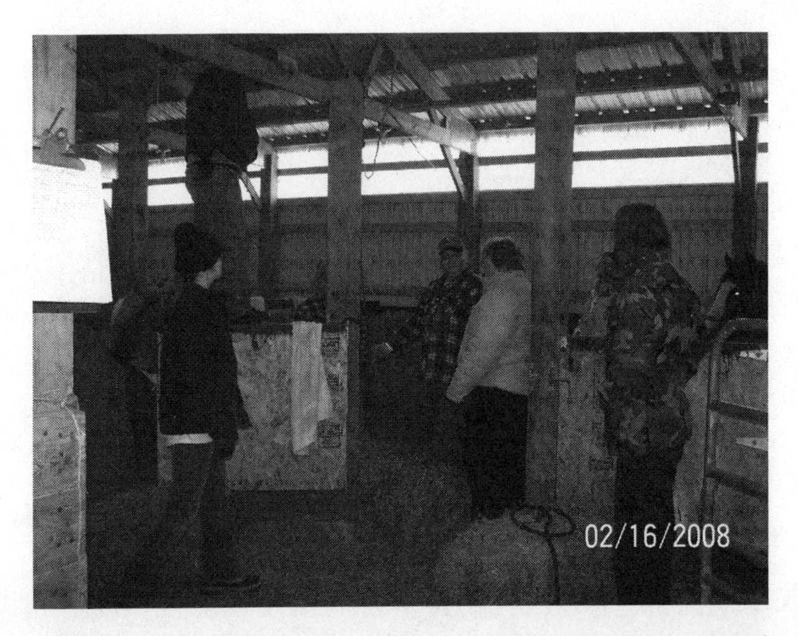

A team of volunteers including Douglas County Sheriff's Department personnel strings the ropes and equipment to lift Windchill to his feet (photo by Jeffrey L. Tucker)

loaded a frozen colt in our trailer, we knew we were facing a life-or-death battle with very little chance of survival. I figured we were in it alone. I could not have been more wrong.

For the next few days after Windchill's first lift, the high points of Windchill life, and ours for that matter, revolved around getting him upright. Although he was still frustrated he couldn't stand by himself, the daily "raising ceremonies" left him in a feisty mood, sparking that fighting spirit, a key factor to his recovery. The stream of visitors and well-wishers continued. This attention also helped tremendously in the spirit-upkeep department. It was during these visits he showed why he was so loved. Without fail, strangers knelt as soon as they were next to Windchill, so they could be closer. Only a

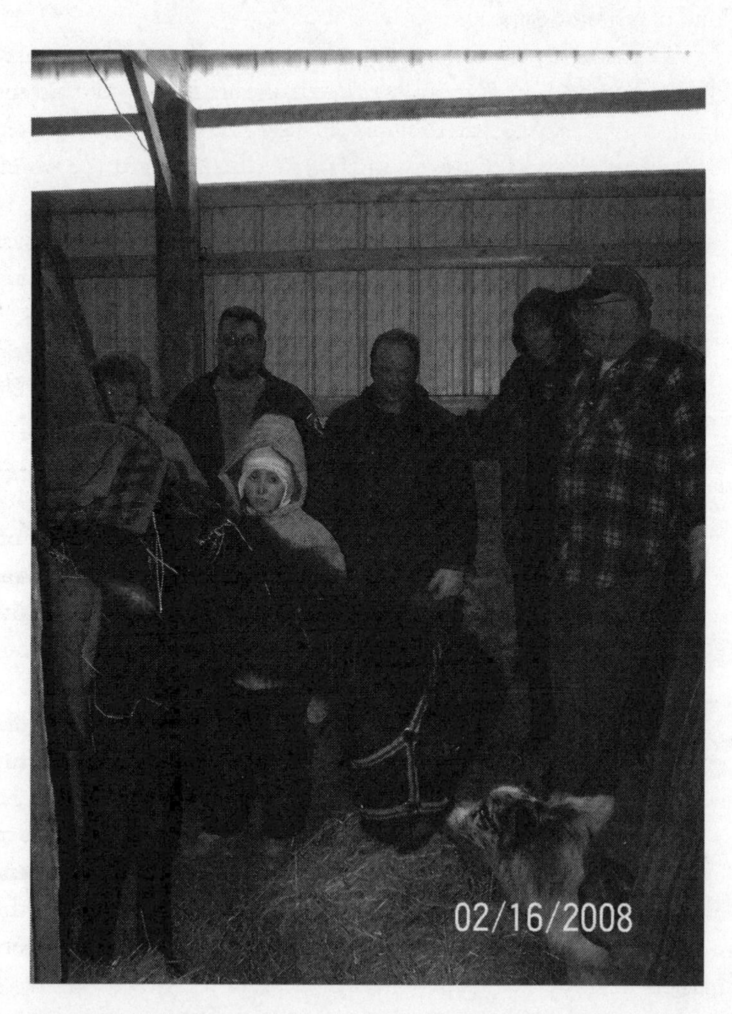

An excited Walker greets his friend Windchill, who stands for the first time in seven days (photo by Jeffrey L. Tucker)

gentle animal who truly wants to be loved consistently inspires that kind of response in people.

His lifts were progressing. He went from twenty minutes to three and a half hours. About midway through one lift, he was taking some small steps when he began to slump. Figuring he was tired, we started lowering him back to the ground. As soon as he heard the winch beginning to move, he immediately sprung back to life, refusing to go down and rest. He was up for another twenty minutes and walked around his stall. He was tired. But his will to stay up and move often overcame his actual energy level.

When he was standing, he transformed from a helpless, sick colt to a show horse. He knew all eyes were on him and people were excited about this progress, and he wanted to please. He nuzzled everyone he passed. He also learned some bad habits from the other horses. Case, one of his neighbors, taught Windchill to chew on his stall door and try to unlatch it. Little things, such as munching on hay and relieving his bladder fully (it just trickled out when he was lying down) were also much easier for him. Draining himself was the first thing he did when he stood. We all cheered, and he looked at us as if we were crazy.

The fact he kept eating was extremely important. He should have weighed 600 to 750 pounds for his age. The vet figured he only weighed about 400. But even at this number, he was a handful to get up, so again, thank goodness for all the good people who came to help. Gary figured out how to rig the chain and winch to the rafters, so that the load was distributed. He later restrung the chains for the winch, giving it more stability and mobility, so Windchill had more room to explore.

One of these expeditions marked a major unexpected milestone. After Windchill refused to be let down and stood for another hour, we finally lowered the sling and realized there was a space between it and Windchill's chest. He was standing on his own the entire time! I had no doubt these miracles occurred because of the thousands praying and hoping on his behalf. His online following continued to grow. Comments from his virtual family and the people who visited in person were so positive, so reassuring, that any chance he would become angry, bitter, or disillusioned due to his treatment prior to coming here was completely eradicated.

When the cold granted us a reprieve at last—temperatures soared to the thirties—and Windchill's strength improved, morale was riding high. Always one for the spotlight, Windchill hammed it up for the TV cameras that came the second week. He was no stranger to cameras. We installed a barn cam, so his online following could see him in real time. It worked fairly well, except in the extreme cold. It could not be on all the time, because it was set up through my laptop, and heaven knows, I can't leave that in the barn all night. If the temperature dropped below nine degrees, it would freeze. Not only would dust and hay wreak havoc with the laptop, but I just knew the horses would be e-mailing in Windchill's name, ordering pizzas, loads of grain, and who knows what else.

Despite all the progress, I was still kind of scared to peek over that stall each morning. Sometimes, Windchill barely moved throughout the night. His position in the morning was often the same as it was when we last left him the previous night, and I would think the worst. Sometimes his hay consumption was down. But I had to remind myself he could not possibly continue eating as much as his first days here. And slowly but surely his ribs were becoming less visible. He also had every right to be so tired that he slept like a rock, not moving much. Still, I was not at ease until I saw him turn his head toward me, which he did every morning after I first looked over the stall door, just as he did to Kathi at every start to her shift.

After proving he could stand for hours by sheer will, he was learning to listen to his body. This is important since most of his

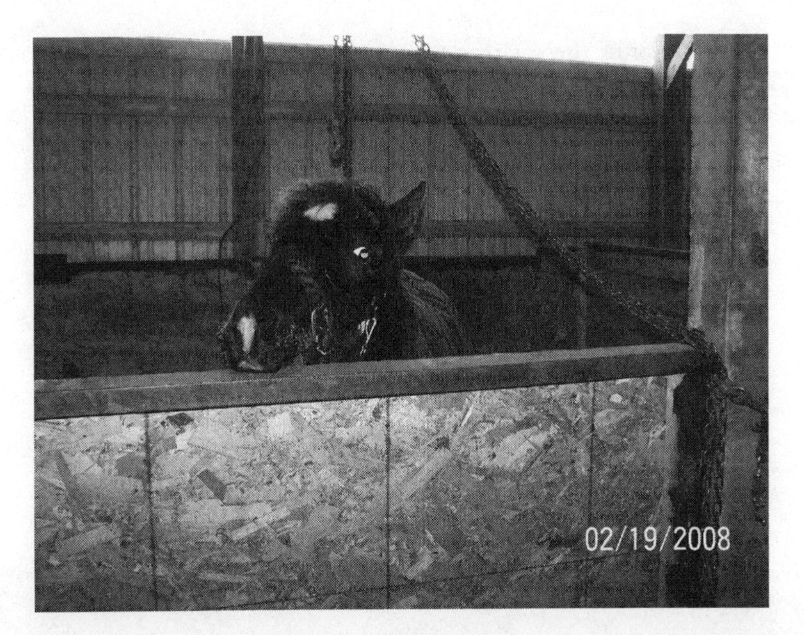

One of the most famous pictures of Windchill, and my favorite; Windchill had stayed on his feet overnight and stood waiting to whinny a "good morning" the next day (photo by Jeffrey L. Tucker)

muscles needed to rebuild completely. At times during a lift, he slowly lowered himself down by his front legs before lowering the rest of his body, when he knew it was time to rest.

But sometimes, Windchill just listened to his spirit. About quarter to seven in the morning on February 19, ten days after Windchill came to us, I made my first check on him for the day. He was still on his feet. That's right: he slept on his feet. His lift the night before began shortly before seven p.m. By eleven he showed no intention of lying down. Too tired to argue, we went to bed figuring he'd come to his senses soon enough and stop refusing to lie down. Ten hours later he was still refusing. There he stood. No sling to support him, just leaning against the stall door.

When people ask me about the spirit of Windchill, I wish they could have approached his stall with me and seen him standing defiantly. It was a picture worth a thousand words.

7

Whirlwind Takes Its Toll

I was beginning to suspect surviving on coffee, cigars, and ibuprofen was not healthy. Kathi was burning through all her paid time off. The lack of sleep and proper nutrition were taking their toll, further intensifying the blur of the life we were living. The constancy of a ringing phone, car wheels crunching down our driveway at all hours, and media interest and inquiries from across the globe were a sort of culture shock. I was starting to understand why Hollywood stars go crazy. We were under constant scrutiny, the subject of public debate, and often criticized. News aircraft circled our residence. People snuck into our pastures trying to get a closer look at Windchill. Some even entered the barn or our pastures when we were out doing chores or at work. The pressure was immense.

Less than two weeks into this, our farm became a tour van stop. One van unloaded members of the Minnesota chapter of the Fans of Barbaro. A passenger walked up to me and asked in all seriousness if she could have anything with my DNA on it. I laughed, but she was not kidding. "A hat, a shirt, anything of yours," she said. "I know I can sell it for five hundred dollars." (I should note that the Fans of

Barbaro have a mission to raise funds to help horses in need so she wasn't asking for personal gain). Another time I stepped out of my house to hear "There he is!" as if it were Oscar night and I had just stepped out of my limo.

These constant visits were not in Windchill's best interest. They tired him out. Always the ham, always eager to please, and always ready for more attention, his outgoing nature kept him from resting whenever someone new was in the barn. The excess attention forced us to institute rules. Our website began listing formal visiting hours, but it did little to stop people from coming whenever they wanted.

Part of the reason volunteers sat with Windchill twenty-four hours a day was concern for his safety. And ours. We got death threats. Windchill got death and kidnapping threats. The original owners and people who boarded Windchill were getting death threats. Some of these crackpots thought Windchill had too much publicity, so it was time to put a bullet in his head. Some were angry, saying we weren't doing enough for him. Others threatened to take him, so we kept our guns loaded and our horse trailers parked to block the gates. We also installed home security web cams.

Windchill's burgeoning notoriety demanded we exploit it, according to a growing number of people. Apparently we were supposed to use our fame and lend our names to this cause or that cause. We heard it at the gas station, the grocery store. The degree to which total strangers felt it was okay to inject themselves into our lives was nothing short of shocking.

Raindance had several horses for sale at the time of the rescue. We could have sold all our horses. Kathi and I decided to place a moratorium on sales, because we were too exhausted to make good decisions and scrutinize potential buyers. We didn't want to rush into a sale and later worry if our horses were in good homes. We made a lot of people angry when we refused to sell. During the rescue, everyone wanted a Raindance horse.

The stress took its toll on my relationship with Kathi as well. With nerves and emotions worn raw and at the surface all the time, seemingly insignificant issues, such as how to spell Windchill, became a big deal. Both of us were running on empty for days, stretched to the point that we couldn't remember if this important task or that everyday chore was actually done. There's a point in exhaustion where the brain flashes for a second suddenly and you realize you're awake, but that your brain went to sleep for a moment. That was happening to me a lot.

Once Windchill emerged from this critical period of recovery, I figured we would actually get to sleep through the night again. It just wasn't possible with a sick "child," especially a child this sick.

The greatest disappointment for me during this critical period was how some supposed animal lovers let us down. When we first got Windchill, we reached out to a major educational institution in a neighboring state known for its equine care facility. Officials there did not return our calls. A local equine organization offered to accept donations on behalf of Windchill. We agreed but never saw the money.

Apparently the director of the neighboring state's university program was friends with the president of this local group, and both wanted control of Windchill, we later learned. These organizations recognized Windchill as a national phenomenon capable of raising significant funds. The school was so territorial, they even told our contact at UC–Davis to stop working with us. Thankfully she ignored them. Dr. Carolyn L. Stull, a nationally known expert in abuse and neglect, had been so generous with her time and advice about how to care for Windchill. She was shocked at the other school's lack of professionalism. "This little horse is more famous than Barbaro, and we want him," they told her. I guess that explains why they never returned our calls. The university would later tell us that while their records did show our calls to them, they were not able to explain why the calls requesting advice were not returned.

Regretfully we did accept the local group's offer to set up a fund for Windchill, since we had nothing in place to handle the volume of donations. We knew the money was pouring in quickly—more than seven thousand dollars in a week—and yet we hadn't seen a penny. Volunteers needed to be compensated for expenses. Costs for supplies and meds for Windchill were adding up. But instead of a check, we got a letter from their attorney, saying we were to correspond exclusively with him.

As expected, the people who had donated to this fund were outraged. We were later told a few board members of this organization resigned in protest. Apparently, much later, the donations were returned to the donors with a weakly communicated rationale that organization leadership did not approve of how we were handling Windchill's care.

We removed all references to this group on our website. Dan's Feed Bin in nearby Superior, Wisconsin, which had already been extremely generous with supplies for Windchill, including giving him the new halter, established a special account for us instead. This account allowed people to donate money for more supplies. Upon hearing of this new fund, the local group withholding our funds was infuriated. They had long coveted the type of exposure our little backyard barn was receiving, but, speaking of barns, not once did they offer one of their heated barns to us. We were told later they feared the presence of a rescue horse might devalue the prized show horses already living there. Amazing.

The course of criticism we got ran from respectful questioning to bitter insult. People wondered why we rehydrated him by holding up buckets of warm water to him, when an IV would work so much better. Or why we didn't just soak him in warm water. They haven't experienced this kind of cold to realize even warm water freezes very quickly in it, and an IV would freeze just as fast.

Some people just flat out told us to shoot him. "He's not worth it," they said. "Why don't you just put him down?" they asked. "What a tremendous waste of resources. Why spend the time keeping an animal alive?"

That certainly would've been the easiest thing to do. Quick and easy—just the way our society has come to expect things. Who will miss an animal, right? I bet even those who suggested he should have "just been shot" (how do you become that callous?) had a pet in their lifetime. I also venture they would have done anything to protect that pet were its life threatened. Perhaps that's why they're so hardened today. Most of us can relate to how a special animal finds its way into our heart. The investment in taking care of our pets produces an incredible return in love, companionship, and adoration. Yet they expect very little in return.

What the more callous commentators didn't realize was that Windchill's story didn't just attract horse lovers. Cat lovers, dog lovers, and animal caregivers from across the globe responded to it. We got a call from a gentleman who cares for gerbils. He wanted to share a few care tips he thought might help Windchill. People who truly love animals "got" this story; they believed every animal requiring human care deserves somebody who will love them.

So back to all the "whys" we were asked. The answers were a series of "becauses." Because we had to try; because we would want someone to try if we were in the same awful circumstance; because humans had put him in this position, so it was our duty as humans to try and get him out of it. Because he was as much one of the Lord's beings as any one of us. I think someday we will, in part, be judged in how well we treated the creatures God entrusted us with. It's a measure of who we are.

To them I asked, "So why is he still with us? His experience with humans up until Raindance had been one of neglect, loneliness, and near starvation. Until then he had only clung to life, never experiencing it in a positive way. He didn't ask to be born. He didn't ask to be starved nearly to death. Maybe somewhere deep in each being's heart and soul is a belief that it can be loved, and that's what Windchill was holding onto."

He devoured the hugs, pets, kisses, massages, and reading and singing to him. I believe he felt in his soul the warm wishes and prayers of the many who reached out to him and wanted him to live. He never had that before. So when I watched him relearning to use his legs, I figured out what he held onto in that pasture as life slowly slipped away from him. It was hope.

So despite the doubters, the critics, the users, and others who wished us no goodwill, Windchill put things in perspective for me. My problems paled in comparison to the thought of him lying out there, clinging to a hope it can get better. And in his case, it would get better. We promised him.

8

Riding the Tides with Windchill

After a brief reprieve, the cold was back, sinking to minus fifty-five wind chills at night and spiking our concern that Windchill's system was unable to bear it. His daily care routine continued to consist of pain meds, antibiotics, fluids, hay, and regular bed turns. The lifts assisted his circulation, a great help in this cold. Now that he was standing, the vet checked if his lungs were clear. So far so good.

He continued to occasionally ignore us when we lowered the lift. Lying around for twenty-three hours a day, it was no wonder he tried to stay up as long as possible. Walker slept in the corner of Windchill's stall almost every night. Those two hung out most of the day, whenever Walker wasn't chasing the two-year-olds in the north pasture. He had decided his role was to annoy Windchill back to health by constantly licking him. Since Windchill responded by extending his legs to push him away, it actually did result in excellent physical rehab. But we didn't tell Walker that he was good for Windchill. He was already long on attitude, short on humility, and emerging as a worldwide sensation.

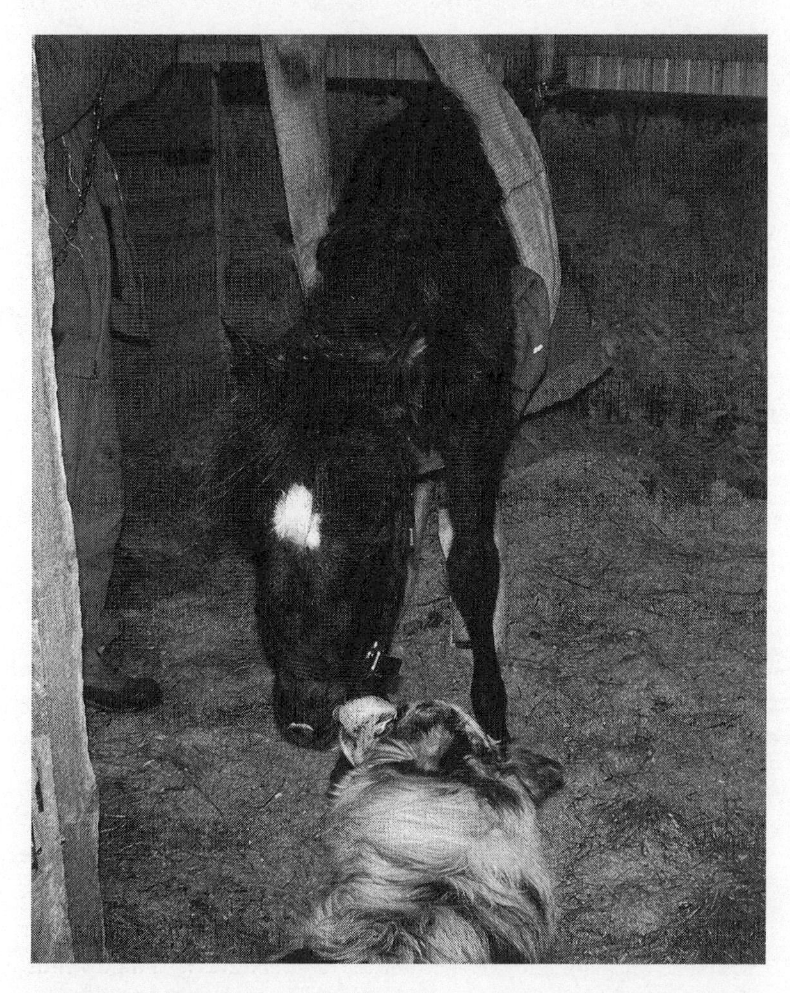

Walker gives his good friend Windchill a kiss on the nose (photo by Jeffrey L. Tucker)

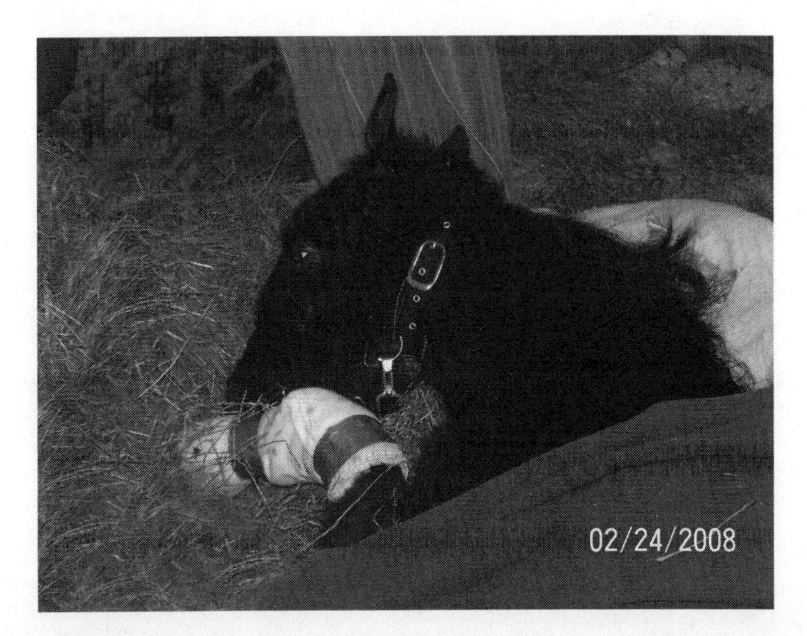

Windchill rests on a bed of straw (photo by Jeffrey L. Tucker)

About a week after his arrival at Raindance, we learned there were no signs of damage from frostbite, which, given his level of exposure when we found him, was amazing. My first thought when hearing the news was of an e-mail from one of Windchill's fans. The gentleman who wrote it said that even if the humans at that farm hadn't paid attention to Windchill's deteriorating condition in that pasture a week ago, God did. No argument here. Windchill's skin, as I said, was paper-thin when we found him. If God wasn't watching over him when he lay frozen in those bitter temperatures and high winds, then why wasn't he frostbit? Our veterinarian said Windchill's case was one of the two worst cases of neglect she had seen in her twenty-year career. Windchill had a purpose. Of that I'm absolutely certain.

Some volunteers feared Windchill was dying. It was a reality we all had to keep in front of us. During the high morale moments, such as his first lifts or recent progress in pushing himself up, that reality got behind me. Then I'd crash with worry. His ups and downs had a profound effect on me. Before all this, I thought I had better "walls" in place, that I could remove myself emotionally when necessary. But since his spirit was so contagious, I couldn't distance myself from it. So whether he was riding high or tired and down, chances were, I felt likewise.

Those of us who were with Windchill every day knew what he was up against. I was beginning to suspect, however, the outpouring of support from hundreds, sometimes thousands of people a day, was springing from a near universal belief that if he had come this far, he had to make it. How I wished it were that easy. Folks would see a newspaper photo of him standing and assumed, "Oh, he's fine now." What they didn't see were the twenty-three hours that he was down, the every six hours he had to be rolled over, or the help he needed to drink or eat. But we clung to the fact that he was, despite severe malnutrition, in stable condition (no pun intended). He shouldn't have been, but he was. His care experts agreed it defied explanation.

The health of a horse's body is rated one to nine on the Body Condition Score. One is completely emaciated. Nine is obese. I thought Windchill would register at least as a one. He was at zero. I took to my laptop, where every raw emotion I felt toward the people who forced this on Windchill fired my fingers across the keys. He was at zero *after two weeks of graining, feeding, and watering.*

February 26, 2008, Blog Entry:

After two weeks of not even registering I have to really, really, really restrain myself from editorializing about how somebody could watch a being literally fade away by starvation like this. I'm not going to tell Windchill his score. We're going to keep telling him he's doing great. The reality is he is a live spirit in a basically dead body. There are probably all kinds of spiritual or clinical experts who could philosophize about how or why the little guy is even still here. I believe hope and an absolutely unfathomable desire to live kept him alive in that cold pasture—a fight that began long before we arrived to drag him out that day.

To the people sniping on the forum, "Why bother? Why save this one horse?" I would ask they come out here and look into Windchill's eyes. The eyes are what capture people's hearts. They shine. They hold wonder, sadness, intelligence and love. I'm not making that up because I'm one of those over-the-top "horse people." Non-horse people have been out to visit in droves and they see him, they kneel by him, and he touches them with his innocence and fierce desire to see all this through. It's not an in your face sort of thing. It's more powerful than that. It's his quiet determination to keep breathing.

Think about it—Windchill didn't suddenly starve. It's a process that takes time. He had to stand out in subzero temperatures and actively decide not to give up—not to do what would have been so easy and so understandable and just lie down and let the sweet release of the bitter cold overwhelm him into oblivion. Another lost soul the world would never have heard of. Instead he went through hunger pangs every day as his body withered away and he felt the signs of dehydration and starvation taking their toll. And he stood out there and waited and hoped and slowly died but absolutely refused to give up until approximately 10 a.m. on February 9th. And even after he had fallen—Windchill REFUSED NOT TO LIVE! That incredible little spirit and your prayers and hope keep alive a little guy whose body has told him he shouldn't be. Kind of makes your problems look a whole lot smaller by comparison doesn't it? I know it does mine. He is completely focused on two things: Living and standing up.

I soon learned sharing my anger and frustration at this raw a moment had consequences. Death threats against the farm owner who had boarded Windchill escalated that day. I realized my writings to Windchill's online fans affected them profoundly. I learned I needed to be careful. My anger about his abuse and neglect spread exponentially to the thousands reading my words. Thus, I learned to be careful in venting my frustrations.

Despite the zero rating, our vet assured us he was making slow progress. He was alive, his eyes brighter, his coat shinier. The fact he stood regularly astounded the vet. But not registering after two weeks was deeply worrisome.

Instead, he had endured hunger pangs every day for months as his body withered away from dehydration and starvation. He had stood out there, waited, hoped, and fought his fate, steeling his neck and pushing it into the wind with every ounce of energy left. After two weeks of registering zero, only an incredible spirit, the power of prayer, and unrelenting hope could keep a body like his alive.

We didn't keep him alive for us. We kept him alive because he chose to live. His bright clear eyes burned that message into our hearts every day.

A few people did not shy from telling us Windchill belonged in a professional facility, not in our "un-insulated backyard barn." From the first day of his arrival at Raindance, we considered transferring him to the school's equine facility once he was strong enough. But as I've explained, their interest in Windchill did not appear to be based on his welfare, but their own. Our vet cleared him for travel, and we had enough donations to help cover the costs of a two-week stay. Even if we hadn't, I had charge cards and would worry about paying them off later. Our greatest concern was the impact the stress of moving would have on him. A ride in a trailer would not be easy on his fragile frame. Another worry was how he slipped in and out of depression. Even though he would be surrounded by equine care professionals, it wouldn't be us, those who had become his family.

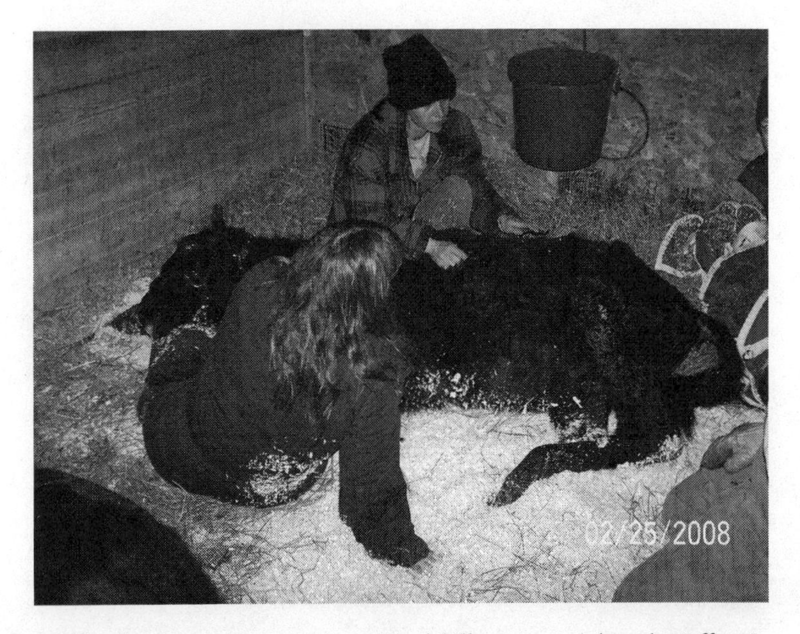

Kathi and a volunteer sit and keep Windchill company (photo by Jeffrey L. Tucker)

The question of whether or not to move him was on everyone's lips, so we decided to consult with our contact at UC–Davis, Dr. Stull. It was her opinion that the stress of moving Windchill might be too much, and the loss of continuity of care might pose an even greater strain. Impressed by his progress, she recommended he stay.

Thank goodness, because I was losing what little sleep I got worrying about a move. I doubted he would be getting the bedside manner he received here, a level of love and attention that I think heals more than any high-tech facility ever could. He was monitored by frequently visiting medical professionals, who were routinely updated by us. He passed his blood work and lab tests with flying colors, so we knew much of his system and digestive tract were fully functional. For a while longer, at least, Raindance would continue to be his home.

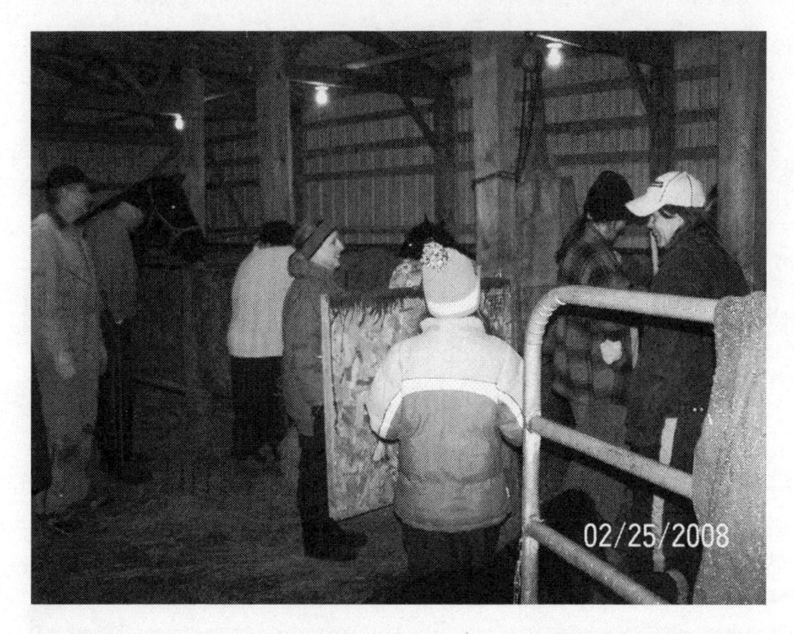

A typical evening in the barn with volunteers and the nightly lift team talking and laughing (photo by Jeffrey L. Tucker)

After the mad rush of the first few days—determining care, finding help, getting the word out, and managing the many donations of hay, alfalfa, blankets for Windchill, and supplies for us, including cookies, hot cocoa, and coffee—routine began to set in. The daytime volunteers reported Windchill was in good spirits. We credited that to the quiet. During the day, there were usually only one or two people with him. In the evening, it was a barn full with more people there to help with his lifts.

If not for the incredible sincerity of concern from his online fan base, I doubt I would have posted all those updates. I fell asleep while writing. I mixed up dates and repeated posts, but averaging three to four hours of sleep, I guess that was to be expected. It was an honor when people told me they started and ended their day with my updates. The depth to their caring kept me going.

After deciding to keep Windchill here, the ups and downs continued. He got so excited about being hoisted up, but lacked the strength sometimes to stay up more than fifteen minutes. Another forty-five minutes would pass, and he started insisting he get another chance. It was like watching a boat adrift at low tide, waiting for the next rush of water to bring it all the way home, all the way to shore. Windchill's shore was standing, and having to lie down meant he was adrift, frustrated at having to wait.

He moved and flexed his legs quite a bit, but they were still cold. Polly, a volunteer, made insulated leg wraps for him, and we changed them often. He moved a bit slower at times, probably due to stiffness from being down so much and the meds. Oh, how he loved those—the powder supplements we put in his grain. He kept sending them back with the waiter. But the little guy desperately needed to rebuild muscle mass, so we were right back at his table refusing to take no for an answer. One of the toughest challenges Kathi initially encountered when he came here was administering any meds that would need to be injected where there was no muscle. Muscle had withered away to skin over bones.

It broke my heart to see how badly he wanted to stand but couldn't always stay up for long. But still, every morning, he nickered "good morning"—a beautiful sound in the quiet of a pre-dawn barn. He continued to rest under his favorite red blanket. He ate and drank. And when I came home from work, Windchill heard me enter the barn and tried to stand by leaning on a hay bale, all the while calling me. Sometimes, his whinny was so loud I could hear it from the driveway.

The hours away at work allowed me to realize when I returned how much he was filling out. Groans and grunts during lifts were getting louder, so I knew I was not imagining this new heft—he was getting harder to lift! He started moving his legs so well I anticipated he would stand on his own soon. He even began taking himself for walks around the stall by pushing himself up against either the hay bales or stall walls and sliding along the perimeter. It was great leg-development exercise. He was standing taller, too. A final sign he was no longer that poor creature we found out in an icy, barren pasture was his brilliant coat. He was so proud of it. After a long brushing, he would look around the barn as if to declare, "Okay, I'm ready for my close-up."

Every day began with uncertainty. Will Windchill stand today? Will he lapse back into a defeated state? Will his legs feel less cold? Will he just want to sleep all day? But as each evening passed into night, we felt like we were given a gift—one more day with Windchill. We would turn off the overhead stall lighting, leaving only the aisle lights, so the horses could wind down. Volunteers would go home and it was just Kathi and me. We would watch him for a while to make sure he was settling in for the night okay, and then it was lights out except for a night light, leaving six colts and fillies to slumber with visions of hay bales dancing in their heads. We would quietly leave the barn, entrusting the brood to a crabby old lady named Annie, whom we knew would quickly quell any after-hours uprising, and a tired Australian shepherd who set up camp in Windchill's stall each night on a bale of hay in the corner.

9

Hitting a Stride

The river of donations, its current driven by the Raindance website, the news media, and word-of-mouth, never ceased to humble me. Alfalfa bales for Windchill. Pizza, pop, and cookies for the crew. Every day, someone dropped something off. People drove hours to see Windchill and bring something. One day I discovered hot chocolate mix—with marshmallows!—sitting on our doorstep. Others special-ordered shipments of coffee for us. One particularly caring and creative idea sprung from the generosity of Deborah Sprague, an artist from Bend, Oregon. From one of the photos we posted online, she painted two pictures of Windchill and Walker, and crafted a purse with Windchill's image on it. She auctioned these works online, raising three thousand dollars for his care.

Others were doing what they could. A woman stopped in, asking if it would be okay to bring the little guy some carrots. As she was disabled, she could not sit with him, but she wanted to do something. Her visit was exemplary of how people didn't have to be on-site at Raindance day after day to make a difference. Just her coming here lifted our flagging energy. That current of caring thoughts, prayers, and action helped keep him alive, helped keep him afloat. Just like people, Windchill knew surviving life's hardships, setbacks, and pain can be almost impossible without the support and love of others.

So many people volunteered. About fifteen people made up our core crew, which was segmented into three to four teams with specific jobs: stall cleaning, feeding/watering, lap duty, and the lift. The crew just sort of came to be. There was no official declaration: "Okay, you, and you and you—lift crew. Be here at six." After the first lift, the same folks just kept showing up the same time every day, about six p.m., and thus, we had a lift crew.

I felt guilty at times knowing I could never thank the volunteers enough. I never knew our driveway could hold that many cars without collapsing. Stacy was there every day, without fail. She passed up job interviews to be with Windchill. I wanted to thank everyone publicly, but some volunteers were getting flak from certain factions for helping us, so I needed to protect everyone's privacy by keeping the volunteer list quiet.

The Raindance farm website hosting Windchill's blog surpassed 2.1 million hits, averaging between 71,000 and 100,000 hits a day. People actually phoned the farm if I didn't update it for a while. With this kind of traffic, it was no surprise some of the input was less than constructive. Despite having no actual physical contact with Windchill, some people were certain they, and they alone, knew what was best. I've always appreciated the opinions of others, respecting and valuing their input. But in Windchill's case, that's where it stopped. What some wanted for Windchill was not only logistically impossible but also possibly life threatening.

What many people failed to understand was Windchill was sleeping in a barn peacefully on a thick bed of sawdust and straw. He was covered in blankets that we rotated and washed several times a day. No, he was not, as some of the blog comments demanded, enjoying the heated barns of polo playing ponies. Polo pony owners neglected to offer us use of their barns or lifts. The only offer we received from another farm was for the lift. And that came from a small dairy and horse farm, where, I'm betting, caring is in far greater supply than money. But he had love, shelter, constant monitoring, and good medical care. Even if money were no object, Windchill was simply too frail to be moved.

Some people were not happy with this scenario, claiming someone other than Kathi and I should have been making decisions regarding Windchill's care. While Kathi had almost a lifetime of caring for horses—including rescue horses—I was a relative newcomer. Unfortunately for them, I'm just a guy who loves horses. I'm not a horse expert. So as a relatively uncomplicated cowboy who enjoys cigars; loves the smell and sound of his fifty horsepower diesel steed "Excalibur" as it carries hay bales to the pastures (the herd considers this their very own "Meals on Wheels"); drives a pickup; listens to country, classical, jazz, and big band; still thinks the Partridge Family might make a comeback; says grace, sir, and ma'am; believes in this great nation and God; and has a dog for a best friend and the three brightest, most talented kids on earth, I was not asking people to believe everything we did regarding Windchill's care was perfect, but to respect that we were doing our best.

E-mails requesting visits were another constant. We had to schedule visitors during the week, so Windchill was not overwhelmed by attention but getting adequate rest. Saturdays were open to everyone—no reservations required. But Sundays the barn had to be closed to visitors. When folks visited, we told them the barn was similar to a hospital room or nursery, so indoor voices only please. Children especially required reminding to walk and talk calmly in the barn area. Everyone wanted to feed Windchill, but we had to monitor his diet carefully. However, with nineteen other horses here,

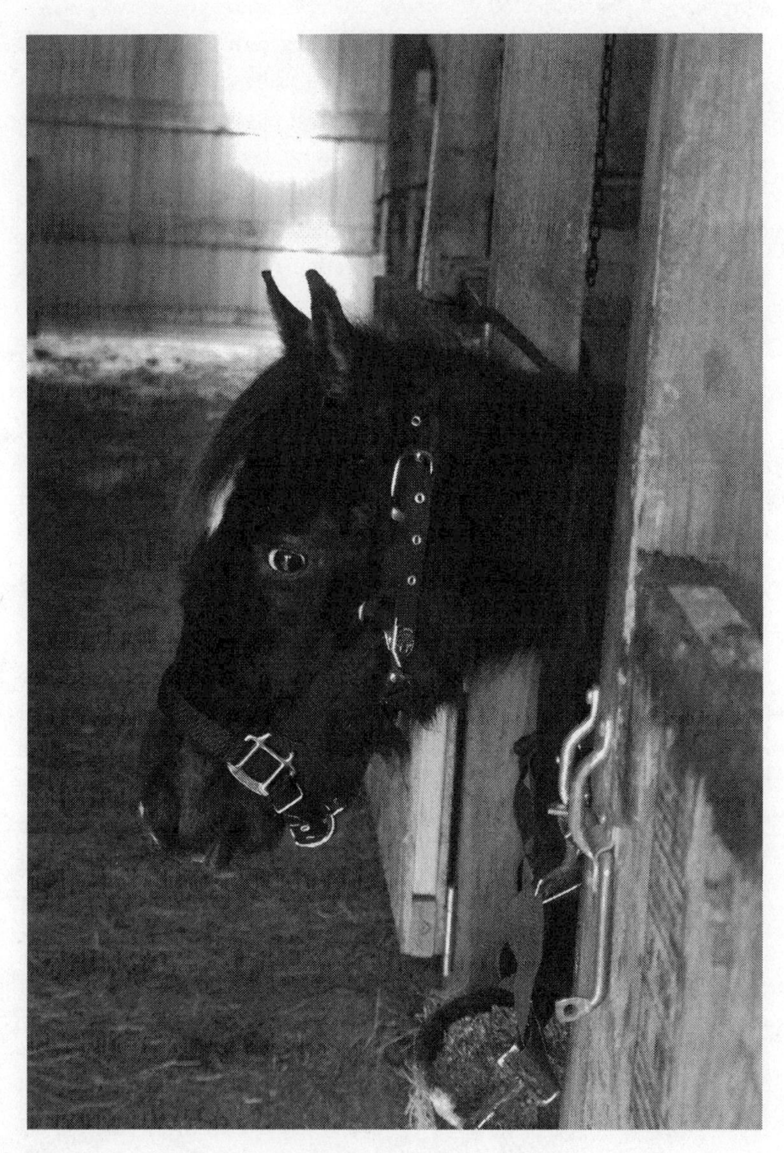

Windchill peeking out of his stall (photo by Kris Bresnahan)

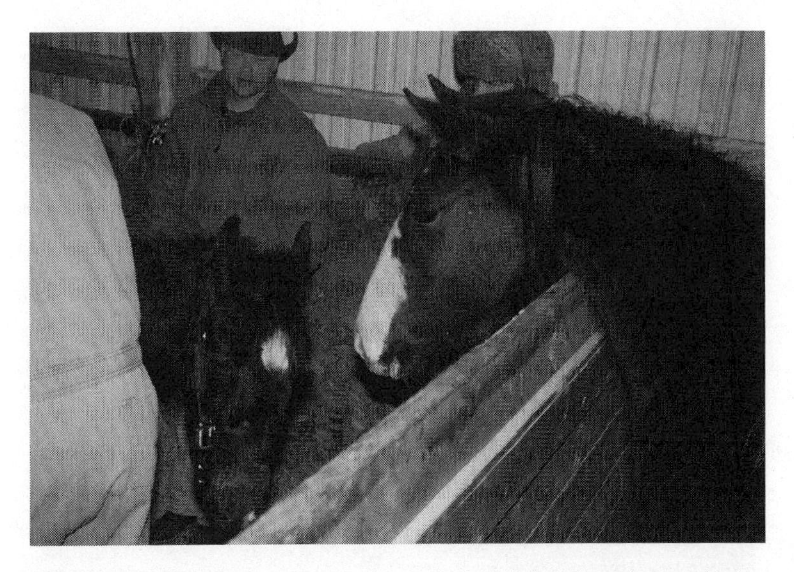

Windchill and his good friend Kisses play as I look on (photo by Kris Bresnahan)

there were plenty of opportunities to pet and feed a horse, not to mention our dog, Walker, and cats Max, Tiger, Olivia, and Cookie, the baby of the cat "herd."

Evidence of forward motion for Windchill was found in looking at photos taken over the course of the first two weeks here. When comparing his coat from the first day to fourteen days later . . . it was not even close. When lobbying for Windchill's Law months later, the condition of his coat when we found him was part of my testimony. I described it as a thin rug of hair over bones. Replacing it two weeks later was a brushed-to-a-sheen, almost plush layer of hair that was smooth to the touch.

Meanwhile, Windchill had some great lifts. He struggled sometimes, because the meds made him groggy. But often he would stand immediately after the initial hoist and commenced to mosey back

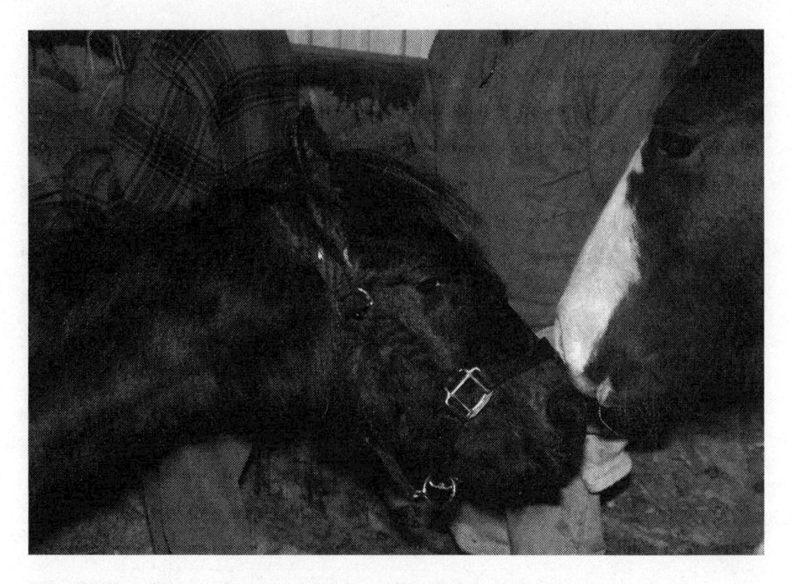

Windchill and Kisses nuzzle across the stall wall (photo by Kris Bresnahan)

and forth between stall walls to say "Hi" to Kisses and "Hello" to Sunday—other young horses. Sometimes we celebrated with pizzas and pop. Windchill would enjoy a new mix of hay that he loved.

We were looking at the before-and-after photos during one such celebration, when I glanced up to see him nuzzling with Kisses. Of course, I didn't have a camera to capture that moment, but fortunately Kris Bresnahan was there later during a similar moment and had her camera. I'll never forget that image or others, such as Windchill seriously into his munching. He would be too focused on hay to nicker a hello, just like a kid too engrossed in a movie to acknowledge Dad when he gets home from work. That was Windchill. If he had a good bale of hay next to him, he was completely oblivious to the crew scrambling around to roll him over, slide new wraps under him, swap blankets, and so forth. We could roll him completely over and he'd never miss a munch. After one of these pizza parties, he usually surrendered to sleep fairly quickly. His quiet breathing always calmed my anxiety about his future.

Life as we knew it became so back-burnered, the burner went out—literally. We ran out of fuel oil in the house. We were so focused on Windchill that everyday tasks had gone by the wayside. I joked with the Windchill blog readers that morning that I was heading outside to warm up. At least out there it had soared up to zero!

Windchill's best friend, Case, had to leave for his new home in Mankato, Minnesota. Windchill still had Kisses and Sunday as neighbors, though, and to cheer him up, we gave him an extra serving of his favorite treat: strawberry yogurt. We never told him he was actually under doctor's orders to eat it, since he needed its enzymes for his stomach. We feared if he discovered yogurt was good for him, he wouldn't eat it. At this point he was up to a one on the starvation measurement scale. The more sources of calories, the better.

The lift crew had worked together so much it was like a well-oiled machine. As UC–Davis advised, we turned him over twenty minutes before a lift to boost his circulation. Then, as Windchill was carefully lifted, the crew turned and balanced him until his legs were under him, and suddenly, we had liftoff. We always had to watch him. Some nights he felt like he was about to make a break for it, and sure enough, there he went, making a beeline for the open stall door. He always munched when he was airborne and got a massage and a good brushing. This lift was one of those when he refused to go down to sleep. And refused. And refused. It was lights out, and the barn went quiet, but Windchill stayed up.

Finally, after thirty hours—thirty hours!—he let us lower him and rested. I fully expected him to roll his eyes the next morning when he heard the winch chains and moan, "Not again." Instead, he started making these little puppy noises (a sort of cute, soft whimpering). When he did that, it meant, "I want up now!" Someone was getting stronger. Stronger by the hour.

It was the kind of breakthrough one wanted to shout about from the rooftops, and luckily for us the media's interest had not abated. A reporter from KARE-11 TV news in the Minneapolis/St. Paul area spent a lot of time with Windchill. The reporter even tried to help me get the barn cam up and running while he was here, but to no avail. Although I'm not at ease with these interviews, having never been fond of public speaking, and am not one to watch much television, I developed a new appreciation for these folks. Many who came to the farm or called us to do a story kept calling and visiting. Others called to check on him, even if they were not planning another story at the time. News people have a reputation for being stoic, aloof—distant from the stories they cover. But I learned just because they have to be objective as part of their jobs, that doesn't mean they don't care.

The more press attention, or any attention for that matter, the more Windchill's spirits took flight. "This is one animal that needs people," I thought aloud one day. Now, with a thirty-hour stand under his belt (or harness I should say), hopefully circulation in his legs was nearing normal. In another week, we would be completely in the clear regarding possible frostbite damage. Given his spirit and determination, I had no doubt there would be more lift records smashed. Considering the extent of his barn family, his people family, and his global fan base, moral support was probably enough to keep him on his feet for an entire week.

We were almost twenty days into this and hitting a stride that became a great comfort to me. Days in the life of Windchill closed with one of the most peaceful times for me. Following a lift, some of us remained for coffee and cocoa in the barn. Windchill opted for hay and water. He was so relaxed with people quietly talking around him. I remember feeling that way when I was little, staying at my grandma's cabin. Early in the morning, about the same time I got up now to care for this tiny colt, I would hear Grandma quietly talking to Grandpa as they brewed coffee. The cabin was heated by wood, so the two smells of strong black coffee and wood burning welcomed the rest of us into the day. I hoped Windchill could look back someday with similar memories of being surrounded by the people and a place that made him feel at home.

10

The Bridge

It was midnight, going on day 21, when I went to the barn for my final check. Earlier that night, the care team left early, as Windchill was more tired than usual. After wandering about his stall for a bit he was down and stayed down. Kathi and I sat with him until nine p.m. We left him his usual self, a bit restless, but nickering a gentle goodnight.

The first sign something was wrong that clear, calm night was Walker. He had come outside to greet me. Since Windchill's first night here, Walker had not left his side at night. I had a bad feeling and ran for the barn, threw open the door, and listened. No little whinny. I called to him. No reply.

I approached his stall. My boots echoing off ice cold frozen ground was all I heard. What I didn't hear, what I wanted so terribly to hear, was the exhale of steaming breath in the cold air. But before I placed my hand gently on him, I knew. No heartbeat.

I buried my face in his neck. It was still warm. How peaceful he was. Still under his blankets, head resting on the towels, no sign of struggle. I struggled with telling Kathi or letting her sleep. She awoke to find me sitting on the edge of the bed, looking at her, and she bolted upright.

"He's gone," I told her.

"Where is he?" Kathi demanded, not fully awake.

With death threats part of our new reality, her first assumption was he had been taken. While I explained Windchill was really gone, Kathi quickly realized he wasn't missing and ran to the barn. I followed and started reliving the scene I experienced just minutes before—throwing the door open, calling to him, running to his stall. Holding him.

Kathi confirmed Windchill hadn't suffered. There were no signs of distress or suffering. He passed quickly and quietly in his sleep. His heart finally gave out, too weakened by prolonged starvation to allow any further recovery.

Just that evening, he'd had his weekly checkup and blood work. His temperature and heart rate were normal. He had gained weight since his last checkup. But when a horse loses 50 percent of his bodyweight, his prognosis for survival is extremely poor. The fact he survived as long as he did and as well as he did was truly a miracle and a testament to his sheer willpower. A horse's body in extreme starvation mode and with no other reserves or means of survival will turn to the only available source of protein available: the tissues of its own heart and vital organs. Essentially a horse's body destroys itself trying to survive.

Thus, in the end, we believe Windchill's growing body and weight hit the limit his weakened heart could support and it stopped. It was quick and painless, and Windchill passed in his sleep. While we never wanted him to go, if he had to leave us, this painless passing was probably the best we could ask for—for his sake.

Shortly after dawn, we announced to the world that sometime between nine p.m. and midnight the previous night, February 29, 2008, one of the bravest souls we ever had the honor of knowing

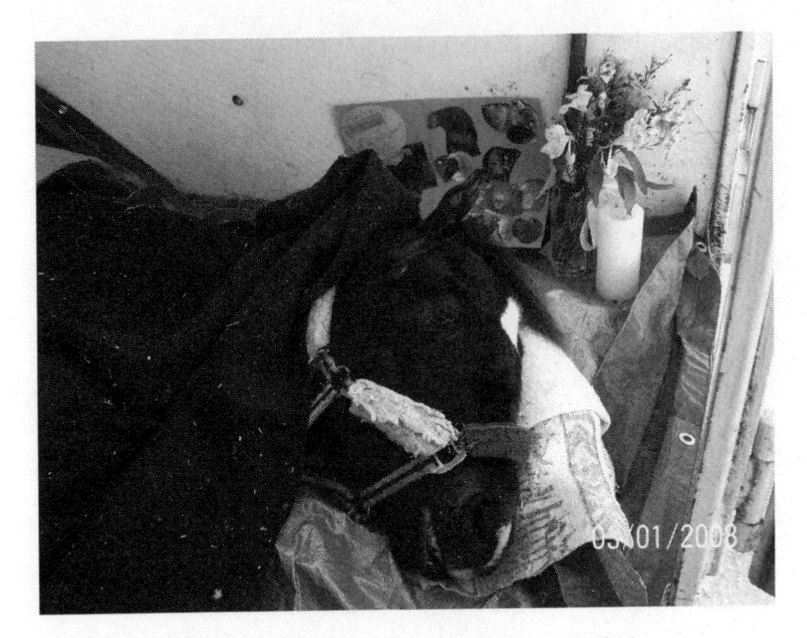

The morning after Windchill's passing (photo by Jeffrey L. Tucker)

crossed over the Rainbow Bridge. He passed quietly in his sleep, surrounded by his two half-sisters, Kisses and Sunday, at the only real home he had ever known.

"There are no words to describe the loss and emptiness we feel," we wrote. Years later, the words still aren't there. My original note was so heart wrenching, Kathi rewrote it.

Experts warned us from the beginning not to get our hopes up, because the odds were just overwhelmingly stacked against him. We never told Windchill that. We accepted each day with him as a gift. We watched his progress in awe, and an entire nation joined us. This little horse became a beacon of hope for so many who had lost their faith in humanity. He taught us that no matter what happens in your life, no matter how unfair, you can still have faith and you can find love to carry you to a better place. He found the good in the world.

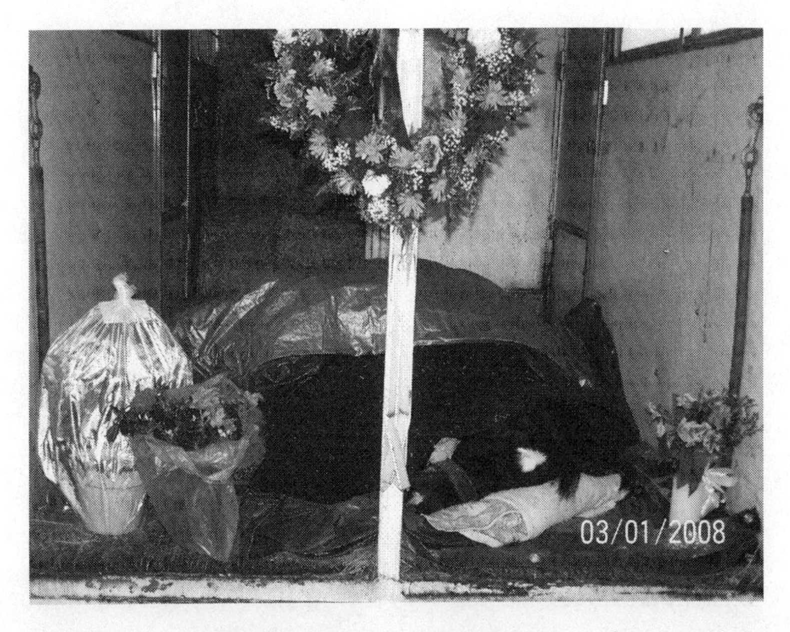

Windchill lies surrounded by flowers that began pouring in from around the country (photo by Jeffrey L. Tucker)

News spread at lightning speed. By eight a.m. WDIO had called. Other media outlets were not far behind. That morning was an exercise in reliving grief. Over and over people came to see Windchill as they have every day since his arrival here. Over and over we had to report he passed away the previous night. Without fail, the news was met with tears and hugs.

His care team arrived early to be with him. They were planning to do a lift that morning and prepare for a pizza party on Sunday. For one last time they gathered together to gently lift him—this time to an empty trailer. Kathi had to leave. I thought I could help but quickly learned I could not. My own pain was so overwhelming. Reminiscent of that drilling wind on the day I first saw Windchill, it took my breath away. Any words of comfort I could offer others went with it.

Ironically, Kathi and I were planning on telling the crew that weekend that it was time for Windchill to leave Raindance. We knew the volunteers were physically and emotionally maxed. None of us could continue leading double lives: full-time jobs and families by day, and every spare moment for Windchill by night. The death threats and other intrusions were also taking a toll. We had decided Windchill was strong enough to move to an excellent equine hospital in Anoka, Minnesota. Windchill would be in a heated, secure facility, and we could continue to be involved in his care.

I honestly thought the next time Windchill left his stall would be under his own power, probably charging out the door into the aisle as he had tried to do so many times. But instead he had to be carried out of it. As news spread, Windchill's admirers arrived in a steady flow throughout the day, bringing flowers, cards, treats, and love. Some were unaware of his passing, but came out of concern because the webcam was off. Had something happened to Windchill? The reality was that, since the vet's visit the day before was nearly the same time as Windchill's scheduled lift, which corresponded with the time we bring the youngsters into their stalls, the cam had to be shut down or become victim of horseplay. Besides, Walker spends so much time mugging the camera, people hardly got to see Windchill some days, just close-ups of Walker's nose.

In the days following Windchill's death, we decided to allow the *Duluth News Tribune* and WDIO-TV to cover the sort of spontaneous wake that was taking place at the farm. We did this out of respect for the rest of the world that was unable to pay their last respects to Windchill in person, and wanted to see him at peace. Both organizations were very caring, respecting those who came to mourn, shooting pictures only after asking for permission.

The people who were able to make it to Raindance were incredible. The woman who won the painting of Windchill and Walker came to pay her respects. She donated her winning bid amount to

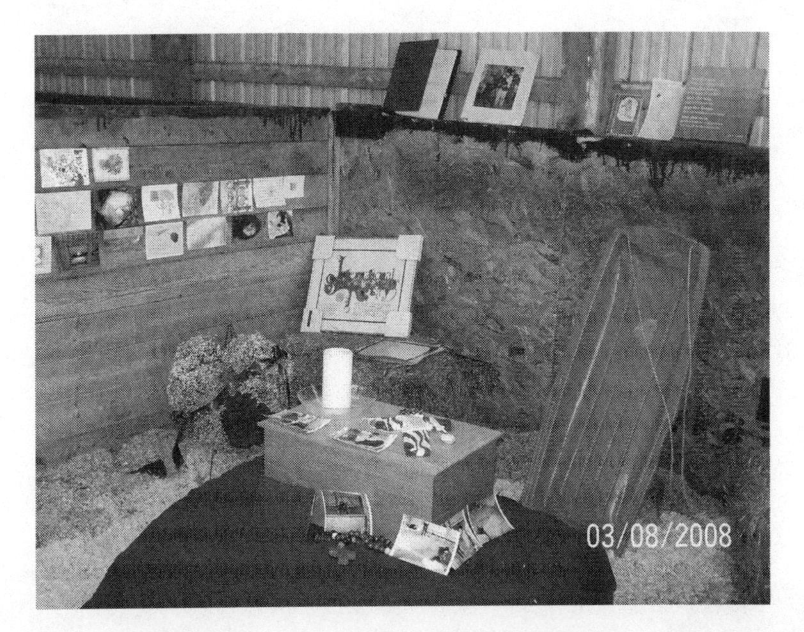

Stall 5—Windchill's stall—set up with Windchill's remains, the orange sled, and pictures and cards that came from all over the country (photo by Jeffrey L. Tucker)

the soon-to-be-created Windchill nonprofit, and generously gave the painting to us to hang above our fireplace. The answering machine filled with messages throughout the day. Many folks were crying so hard, we couldn't understand the words but could fully understand their meaning and sentiment.

The hours wore on. People kept coming. Tears kept flowing. The raw sinking ache inside me kept deepening. But at least the blur of constant interaction kept that ache from consuming me whole. Then seemingly, in an instant, it's all gone. The driveway's quiet. A dull winter dusk shutters the sun. Is that a sliver of pink trying to slip through this pallet of every possible degree of gray? What sunset is Windchill seeing tonight? I think I know.

For several days my mental state swung from coherent thought to eyes burning, sliding into hell. I thought of Windchill and the hell he went through. But he ended up at a better place, our place, our farm, where he was loved. His hell ended and so will ours. Less than four weeks later, Bonnie, one of Windchill's moms, gave birth to Layla. The entire care team was back at the same stall, and I helped with the delivery. I could see Windchill there smiling and watching the new baby.

After towel drying Layla, we wrapped her in Windchill's favorite red blanket. It seemed appropriate, though I had to pause for a moment and turn away. Seeing anything of Windchill's made my heart rain again. But seeing Layla wrapped in that red blanket started filling an emptiness that has weighed me down since losing Windchill. Until that day, the emptiness felt as if it would swallow me whole every time I walked by Windchill's stall without seeing him in there. I'd see him in there walking circles around the stall, smiling with pride. The sight of little Layla brought the first real smile to my face since Windchill died.

We decided to put Kisses back in the stall she had given up for Windchill right away. Since I kept "seeing" Windchill there, pushing himself around with his legs whenever I walked into the barn, having Kisses back in there helped.

The road back to normal life was long. The time we lost, what would normally pass as our lives—sleep, get up to let horses out, go to work long hours, come home to bring the herd in, feed, grain, and water them, crash in a chair for a quick bite to eat and relax—that all became hypercontracted during our twenty days with Windchill. We still had to do all that and care for him. Both of us lost weight; Kathi lost ten pounds and I lost eleven, which I think I could afford, though, so thanks, Windchill. In the days after his death, I finally crashed hard, as the adrenaline that had carried me through those sleepless nights by Windchill's side evaporated in an instant. This was unfortunate, since the adrenaline also masked the fact I had been suffering from walking pneumonia for the last month.

The cost of lost sleep and the toll on our health was a very, very small price to pay for what we wanted to give to Windchill: belief in humans again and the knowledge he could be loved. Windchill gave back so much more. He humbled me to a degree that is difficult to describe. While our lives returned to their previous routine, they would never be the same. Windchill's contagious spirit, his quiet resolve, and that candle of hope inside him is forever lit in us. It was all there in those bright eyes of his. A photographer came close to capturing it and that photo is now the cover of this book.

That first night, I did not go gently into life without Windchill. The only way I could let go was to do so slowly, grudgingly . . . by still hanging on for a while. Hanging on with questions. And I wouldn't let go until I had answers. Or so the grieving mind thinks. For hours after I found Windchill, I searched the Internet, reading everything I could find on horse starvation. Like our kids, beloved pets become a part of you. Because they're innocent, love unconditionally, and expect so little in return, you want to protect them and hold them close.

So I searched for a reason to blame our actions. Was it the care we provided? I guess in my anguish I needed to find something we did wrong, something we should have done, or some miracle cure we overlooked. Six or seven hours later, my eyes were raw and the answers kept coming up the same. They reinforced the overwhelming odds stacked against him and what a miracle it was he lived as long as he did and accomplished as much as he had: standing, walking, and regaining strength and weight. His organs were never going to support his body again. The damage from the starvation was too severe. So to keep living, his spirit had to leave his body behind. By morning, my anger shifted from myself to the people who really made this happen. God, I pleaded, help me to forgive because I'm having trouble doing it myself.

That night, and for the days to come, the only part of the world that kept me sane was a virtual one. I could continue the conversation there. I could escape the quiet. So many cared enough to keep talking, to fill that emptiness, with calls, prayers, e-mails, and posts. It helped that I could leave night's darkness and bitter cold to find warmth online for a brief time before having to go back outside.

It never occurred to me—but then again, little did that first day—that some people may not have understood my announcement when I referenced Rainbow Bridge. Having seen wonders and miracles, and felt the spirits of animals and people alike, I have no doubt there is such a place.

> Just this side of heaven is a place called Rainbow Bridge.
>
> When an animal dies that has been especially close to someone here, that pet goes to Rainbow Bridge. There are meadows and hills for all of our special friends so they can run and play together. There is plenty of food, water and sunshine, and our friends are warm and comfortable.
>
> All the animals who had been ill and old are restored to health and vigor. Those who were hurt or maimed are made whole and strong again, just as we remember them in our dreams of days and times gone by. The animals are happy and content, except for one small thing; they each miss someone very special to them, who had to be left behind.
>
> They all run and play together, but the day comes when one suddenly stops and looks into the distance. His bright eyes are intent. His eager body quivers. Suddenly he begins to run from the group, flying over the green grass, his legs carrying him faster and faster.

You have been spotted, and when you and your special friend finally meet, you cling together in joyous reunion, never to be parted again. The happy kisses rain upon your face; your hands again caress the beloved head, and you look once more into the trusting eyes of your pet, so long gone from your life but never absent from your heart.

Then you cross Rainbow Bridge together . . . (author unknown)

The comments on the Windchill blog almost crashed the server again. A memorial page flew up within hours, and hundreds of e-candles were lit in his honor at gratefulness.com.

Missy in Maine: I am sitting here, sobbing and heartbroken, over the loss of little Windchill. Thanks all of you for giving him the love and care you did, and to your wonderful doggie who stood by. I'm so sorry.

Robin in Pennsylvania: Even though I know Windchill is gone, the first thing I did this morning was check the website and guestbook. I know I will continue to do this for a long time! The connection this little guy brought to us is just incredible. Some people may think we're crazy but we all know the truth. THIS is important. THIS was amazing. And WINDCHILL did it. We can ALL stay connected through the nonprofit, and Windchill's life will NOT have been in vain. Thanks again to all who helped and thanks to those who have written poems and verses in the guestbook. Even though I cry as I read them, they've helped me so much.

Cindy in New York: I didn't get a chance to log on yesterday to see how Windchill was doing and now I'm devastated. I can only say that I have considered it an honor to share his story along with the nation's animal lovers and to root for the most beautiful little colt I have ever seen. I can only say thank you to Jeff and Kathy for sharing their lives with me and opening the doors of their barn to catch glimpses of Windchill's progress. In Garth Brooks's words "I could have missed the pain, but I'd have had to miss The Dance." Rest in Peace.

Renee in North Carolina: Rest in peace, little one. You deserve it. I am sure that Jeff will meet you at the Rainbow Bridge one day. Please look for my beloved Trojan who crossed in December. He will help you if you need anything.

Nancy in Tennessee: I have tried for several days to get through but someone or something is blocking me out. I can't even begin to say how saddened my husband & I are over Windchill's passing. He was like a "Beacon of Hope" in a jaded world. He was something to hold on to, like seeing a light in the sky, a ray of hope. Jeff, you, Kathi, and all of your crew are such an inspiration. I pray that a lot of good will come from this tragedy. Oh how Windchill will be missed. Goodbye, little champion of strength and hope.

Melanie in Minnesota: I just took a quick look online at the barn cam of the North Pasture, and how appropriate, it has raindrops on it. The world's tears . . . Godspeed Windchill . . . We all love you and miss you dearly!

Questions about how to honor Windchill's legacy were also flooding in. We all knew Windchill's place in our lives was not going to go away. In fact, his influence on the world was just beginning.

11

Living the Windchill Legacy

One evening after Windchill died, I was sitting at a stoplight in Superior, and a biker dude stopped alongside me. He looked at the farm logo on my truck and motioned for me to roll down my window. I assumed this was the way I was going to die.

"You're that guy who tried to save that little horse?" he asked.

"Yes, I am," I replied.

"That was righteous, man. I'm sorry he died, but at least you tried."

Then he nodded and roared off.

Many of the people who followed Windchill's story told me they never thought they would become so riveted by something like this. They didn't understand why they attached immediately and deeply to this little colt and stayed that way until the end. I think the reason has something to do with the fact that they saw what we saw in the barn. Despite the odds, despite the terrific sadness accompanying his first nine months of life, his last twenty days proved people can take amazing steps to help another living being overcome those odds and erase that sadness.

For many days after Windchill's death, my post office box was full. There was always a note to go to the counter. "Oh yeah, you have a ton of mail," was the usual comment from the postal clerk on duty when I presented the card. It's a good thing my truck has an extended cab. I needed it for the cookies, care packages, other gifts, cards, and pictures drawn by kids for the Windchill crew, as well as donations for a Windchill nonprofit. In the spirit of the Appaloosa part of Windchill and Native American tradition, a local woman sent a pouch with tobacco to keep near Windchill's urn. The Fans of Barbaro registered a star in Windchill's name, appropriately in the Pegasus cluster, and sent a beautifully framed declaration.

The first grade class from Meadowvale Elementary School in Elk River, Minnesota, sent a scrapbook they created in Windchill's honor. Ms. Millard's class included a poem so lovely, it reminded me wisdom is not exclusive to older folks.

Someday . . .

Someday . . . Windchill you will prance in the tall grass—Charlie
The sun will warm your shiny coat—Kylee
You will lift your head up high—Tyler
Someday . . . you will meet up with Case again—Kayden
Someday you will race with your friend Case—Peyton
Someday you will eat like a horse—Elana
You will tell your story to new ponies and the cats in the stable—Sophia
Kisses and you will walk in the fields of clover—Sarah
Someday . . . you and Kisses will eat that clover yum!—Cole
Someday . . . you will remember all the love—Gracie
You, Windchill, are love!—Caleb
Someday . . . you will read our book at bedtime—Drew
It will help you sleep tight—Aaron
Do you get hot chocolate? you should!—Preston

Someday . . . you will be big and strong—Dylan
Someday . . . you will hear the rain and feel cozy—Riley
You will jump up high and kick up your heels—Marlena
The thunder is just a loud noise, it won't hurt you like the cold—Sam
You'll call out really loud, because you are happy—Kate
Someday . . . you'll give out your autograph hoof—Alicia
You're famous Windchill!—Anna
Someday your pretty legs will hold you again—Evan
So you can have fun all day!—Blake
Someday . . . you will feel well again—Kelli

To say this experience has changed my outlook on life may sound cliché, but moments such as the exchange with the biker at the stoplight awaited me around many corners. People were stopping me all the time to offer condolences, thanks for our efforts, and so forth. Others e-mailed saying they couldn't stop crying. During my time in the Air Force, I was once at the end of a runway when an F40 fighter started moving out of position, with me failing to notice. I turned around to find myself looking into the turbines as the pilot wound it up to taxi. The force of air inflated my lungs, picked me straight up, and I flew upward in a perfectly vertical position. This lasted for several seconds before I landed on my feet. That feeling was nothing compared to what I have experienced from the power of the love and caring from the Windchill faithful. It was awesome, and I had boxes of coffee and cookies for weeks to prove it.

Windchill taught me how one step does matter. The world changes in steps. I'm positive that his spirit and memory have showed thousands, if not more, that someone can change the world one step at a time. I have grown more certain of that with each day that has passed since he left.

In retrospect, Windchill's legacy started with the first ring of the phone on February 9, 2008. That call asking us to check on a downed colt started a movement to declare war on equine neglect. Throughout the commentary on the Windchill blog during those twenty days, the idea to create a nonprofit in his honor was broached numerous times. Within days of Windchill's funeral, the idea for the WindChill Legacy Ltd. was formed. Within a couple weeks it had a board of directors, of which I served as president. Within a month, we had a mission statement, born from the dialogue on the blog.

Kathi and I hadn't been able to decide on the spelling of Windchill's name. She preferred two words, with the "c" capitalized, so we compromised with "WindChill" for the name of the nonprofit, and I kept it lowercase when writing about him. It seems unique, more personal to me. By the end of 2012, the foundation had officially changed its name to the Windchill Legacy Ltd., with the lowercase "c."

The nonprofit's mission encompasses several goals, including stopping situations like Windchill's before they happen. We wanted to start a fund to assist with gelding stallions. Working with veterinarians, we wanted to stem the problem of unplanned, and often unwanted, foals. We've made some progress on this front, primarily working with individual farms. Equine abuse manifests in many ways. Some farms raise more horses than any small farm ever should, only to sell most of those horses dirt cheap to pay for feed for the others. "Senseless" doesn't begin to explain this practice or this type of horse breeder. In addition to working with area farms, the Windchill Legacy has donated to gelding programs.

Another way to stop these situations before they can start is to educate people, especially the young, about proper care for all animals, not just horses. We began preparing presentations and programs for schools, 4-H clubs, senior citizen homes, and other organizations. We also thought it might help make the story of equine abuse and neglect more real if somebody who had actually lived the story was the one to tell it.

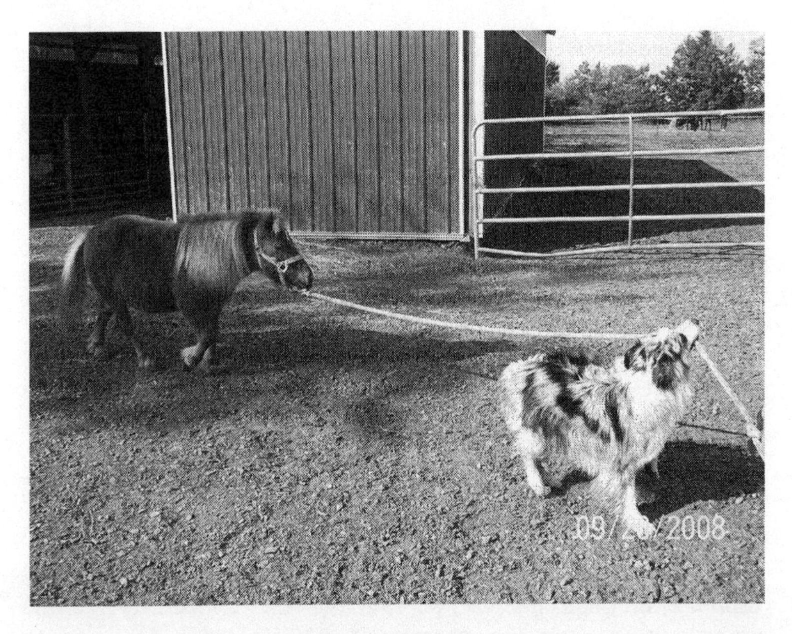

Walker walks Magic, a miniature horse that was utilized to bring the Windchill message to schools and nursing homes around the region (photo by Jeffrey L. Tucker)

In September 2008, a miniature horse by the name of Magic the Mini arrived at Raindance. Magic knows all about equine rescue. Raised on a miniature horse breeding farm, Magic was severely neglected. Magic was of no value to the farm, because she could not get pregnant. The woman who rescued Magic found the horse knee-deep in mud and looking absolutely miserable. Magic had never been brushed or handled much at all. The poor horse flinched every time someone tried to touch her.

The summer after Windchill's death, Raindance Farms held its First Annual Windchill Barbeque. People who had followed the Windchill story came from all across the country to talk, laugh, cry, and game-plan how to continue his legacy. The woman who had rescued Magic was there.

Magic was soon serving as our new equine education coordinator. Magic the Mini began her first rescue education tour just one month later, in October 2008, by visiting a youth center in Superior. This was the first effort by the Windchill Legacy nonprofit to make our mission public. There were many, many more to follow, and these efforts continue to this day.

One of the Legacy volunteers once commented there was nothing quite like walking down a school hallway with a horse on Iowa Basic Skills Test day. The quiet hallway echo of hooves on linoleum became quickly accentuated with audible gasps, giggles, and whispers of "Did you see . . . ?" Waves and pointing gestures followed us past each door as teachers tried to steer the pencils back to paper. Later when the testing ended, the children filed into a designated classroom for our presentation. We talked about how we found Windchill, showed pictures of him in the barn, answered their questions, and then heard another litany of gasps when I told them Windchill died.

The Legacy crew was worried about this, but the teachers assured us the children could handle it, and they did. One girl shouted, "He is in horse heaven now!" Other kids talked about their own pets passing away. I listened to each child who lost an animal and offered my condolences. On a more uplifting note, the children then turned to Magic for pets and hugs, and we talked about her happy ending—the kind we want for every rescue.

This type of day has repeated over and over as the Windchill Legacy's education team has visited schools, Boys and Girls Clubs, and other youth groups across our area since Windchill's death. In just one year, Magic logged 1,698 miles conducting 34 outreaches, 17 of them in schools (33 classrooms total), 13 of them in nursing homes and assisted living centers, 2 to special interest groups, and 2 promotional events. A total number of 3,164 people were reached.

When Legacy volunteers took Magic to visit facilities for seniors, the experience resembled what happens with school children. As soon as the seniors or the children would see Magic, they wanted to touch her, pet her, give her a hug. Both groups would smile with delight when seeing what was on her head—a tiara. It helped get Magic in the zone: "The queen is now granting audiences," she seemed to neigh as soon as we put it on. Upon entering a home, we cleared out the salon almost every time. The ladies couldn't take their hands off Magic. Within minutes, she would be the one getting the full treatment—brushing, braiding, beadwork for her mane, massages. They would have done her hooves if we had the time. Magic was eyeing the fuchsia polish during one makeover.

Magic has since retired from the Windchill Legacy, and new minis are now taking her place. But when Magic was on duty for the Legacy, she lived up to her name almost every time. There were moments of breakthrough that touched everyone who witnessed them. A gentleman staying in an Alzheimer's unit fell in love with Magic. He had been around horses in better days, and Magic could sense this. From his chair, he pulled Magic's halter and brought her face closer to him. All of a sudden, he broke into the biggest smile and he started talking to Magic. He started talking to us—in clear sentences. His daughter was there visiting, and her eyes grew wide as she told us he had not smiled for a long, long time, let alone have a conversation. He talked about his time with horses, telling stories his daughter had never heard before. "Someone trained this horse right," he told us. While we beamed, his daughter put her arm around him and laughed. It was a different room than the one we first entered a half hour earlier.

Bringing a horse into a medical facility was actually nothing new for me. My grandma, one of the greatest people I have ever known, wanted to meet Rain, my first horse. It was important to her to see Rain, because Rain was a part of me, but she was living in an assisted living facility at the time. She asked me repeatedly to find a way to bring the horse to her, so one time I wheeled my grandma out to the curb and there was Rain. I brought Rain to the home several times. Each time the management asked me to please not bring a horse on premises, so I'd wait a while and then do it again. The staff cheered me on. The management hated me. Working with Magic allowed me to honor a promise I made to my grandma to give other home-bound seniors a chance to connect with a living, breathing memory from their past. Magic even visited the very home where my grandma stayed before she passed away.

Thankfully, the people operating the homes we visit realize the healing power these visits have. One resident who was deeply depressed had us in tears after a visit. She was lying in bed when we entered her room, and the second she saw Magic she started crying. Magic came up to her, and laid her head on the woman's bed. More tears. After a few minutes, the woman swung her legs out of bed and one of our team members put Magic's head on her lap. After still more tears and several lunges for the Kleenex box, we heard the woman whisper, "She is something. She is so precious. So calm. You're special aren't you? Stay with me . . ." She then thanked us for bringing Magic to her. We lingered there for a long time. When it was time to go, she had a smile on her face.

These encounters, especially those with Alzheimer's patients, were hard on Magic. We could tell by how she drooped her head and slowed down, as if she couldn't visit one more room. But she almost always kept going. During this same visit we paused by a door to see a woman with her mother, who was ninety-three years old. "Mother will not be here much longer, but please, please come in," the daughter said. We were worried the elderly woman was tapped emotionally, but upon hearing how she had raised horses and been around them all her life while raising eleven children, we couldn't refuse. This woman had grown up on a farm where all the work was done by horses. We walked in, and she was sitting in a chair, covered with a blanket, eyes closed. After sliding furniture aside, Magic was walked to her. The daughter bent down to tell her mom a horse had come to visit. The woman opened her eyes, focused them on Magic, and smiled. Together the daughter and her mom stroked Magic. "I think Magic reminds my mom of her favorite horse, Nellie," she said. "Look," she said a few minutes later, "My mom is getting more alert!" The daughter radiated joy.

We stayed for a while, until her mom closed her eyes again. The daughter then told us how this was the most alert she had seen her mother—how it was the first thing they had connected over—in a long time. Witnessing the love of a daughter for her mother, her gentleness and patience had us tearing up once more.

Another visit to a different facility was made memorable by a woman who, with the help of a walker, made not just one but several treks through the crowd milling about Magic to approach and pet her. I could tell it took tremendous effort for her to get on her feet to make these trips. When she made it to Magic, she didn't want to leave. Later, the administrator told me he had not seen this woman on her feet for months.

The beauty of Magic's visits is how they reincarnated wonderful memories, cherished images from days gone by that might have been lost forever. They are shared with sons, daughters, or other relatives who happen to be in the room for a second chance at posterity. One fellow told us how his sisters and brothers were pulled in a toboggan by horses. Once the toboggan went too fast, and the four of them ended upside down between the horse's legs with the toboggan on top of them. The horse did not move. He said their dad gave them a good talking to about how lucky they were to be alive. Another lady reminisced about a horse in her neighbor's field. She always brought an apple for him on her way to school. That horse waited for her in the same spot every day.

Some of the most bittersweet words I ever heard were spoken by another Alzheimer's patient. In one burst of lucidity, she announced,

"I will always remember this." If only that were true. That same day we visited a quadriplegic who was almost completely immobile. All he could do was move his eyes, and move his head slightly. Magic was tired that day, but she stayed with the gentleman. Her head on his lap, she stayed and stayed. After several minutes the man's face lit up and shone with tears.

If, on February 8, 2008, someone were to have told me I would soon be spending my Friday afternoons escorting small horses to nursing homes, assisted living centers, elementary schools, and community centers, I would have laughed. But this is how I live differently now that I've had Windchill in my life.

One group connected with Windchill's story like no other. Two years after Windchill's passing, we took Magic to a multiple sclerosis support group. People there told us they identify with Windchill because of their disability. His struggles to survive, his will to live, his fight to not give in to the cold—it all rang true with their own experiences of not giving up when diagnosed with MS. Windchill held onto hope out in that field that someone would help him and make his life better. They can relate, as each of them hopes for a cure with each passing day.

One person in the group said, "Windchill in the sling reminds me of all the contraptions I have had to use over the years, to stand and get places." There were a lot of tears and a lot of anger there that day. They were victims of fate, which is bad enough. But how could someone willfully force such a fate upon another being?

In respect to that anger, the Windchill Legacy has been pursuing legislation that is more than a slap on the wrist to those who cause suffering to animals, through either abuse or neglect, although the line between the two is razor thin. The proposed legislation adds "great bodily harm" to the definitions of abuse and provides stricter punishment for clearly identified cases of abuse or neglect. There are tougher laws in other states and we believe there should be a

Windchill's Law in Wisconsin to help protect all animals. We also want to develop resources for those pursuing similar statutes in other states that lack them.

With the help of Nick Milroy, our representative in the Wisconsin Assembly, we introduced Windchill's Law during the 2009–10 session but ran out of time for a full assembly vote. As this book goes to press, the new draft of the law is being presented in committee hearings and continues to gain support.

Another area of focus for the Legacy involves establishing a formal response structure to deal with a case of neglect when it is reported. If a case is confirmed, we want a network of rescue transports ready, that is, people with trucks and trailers willing to assist in animal transport. Sheriffs' departments are not equipped to do this. We also want to develop a network of facilities and volunteers in various locations that would be ready to assist in a neglect case at a moment's notice.

To enhance the effectiveness of this response structure, we also identified development of an electronic resource network as a priority. This would allow a nation of caring people to come together over a common cause. One of the most amazing lessons from Windchill's rescue was how God provides the resources when they're needed, and in our case, he provided them through the electronic "world" of the Internet. When we began to burn out, he gave us wonderful volunteers. When we needed a sling and winch, he brought us the Aho family of Cloquet. Whatever we needed, somebody somewhere had the answer. Most amazing to us was that this happened in real time. We'd post the need online, and it was filled—sometimes within minutes. The Legacy now wants to make that dynamic we experienced with Windchill a permanent resource for equine rescues.

The Legacy has donated books to school libraries and other organizations. It has also raised funds for rescue and gelding programs across the country. The Windchill phenomenon of connecting people with the magic of horses has taken on a more permanent role in some people's lives. A number of people tell me they have finally followed through with a lifelong dream to learn to ride after following Windchill's story. Others started volunteering in animal rescue shelters.

"I knew virtually nothing about horses," wrote John Henderson of Bellevue, Washington. "I knew little about the issue of horse abuse and neglect and the growing problem of thousands of unwanted horses in this country. I wasn't a horse person by any stretch of the imagination, but I had always admired their beauty and grace from afar."

In December 2007 John had lost his fifteen-year-old yellow lab Sadie. He was still mourning her death when one evening two months later, he happened to catch a news story on Fox about this cowboy way out in Wisconsin who had just rescued a nine-month-old colt that was found starving and freezing to death in a local pasture in subzero conditions.

"Something about the man and the story captured my attention, maybe in part because my feelings were still so raw over losing Sadie," said John. "Whatever it was, I went online that night to check out the story and those who were telling it. It turned out to be a story that would change my life forever, and I found a new friend in Jeff Tucker.

"As the days and weeks went by, I became more engrossed in the events unfolding in a stall at Raindance Farms. I read Jeff's blogs every day, sometimes with cheers, other times with tears. I did so until that fateful day of February 29, when it all came to such a gut wrenching end."

John began writing me, expressing both condolences and an acute ability to relate to my loss. We became friends and, in doing so, he got a crash course about the terrible degree to which horse neglect, abuse, and abandonment is a problem in our country.

"What can I do to help?" he asked, and I suggested he research the Bellevue area for horse rescue groups that needed volunteers.

"In short order, I found one called Hope For Horses, just fifteen miles from my home," John reported. "One evening I attended a fundraiser for it to meet the owners, John and Jenny Edwards, and to ask a few questions. We talked for nearly an hour. I told them about losing Sadie, and John had an idea. He asked me to follow him and in his car was the most lovable Weimaraner named Grady, who was immediately all over me. I was grinning from ear to ear."

Soon John was mucking stalls and corrals at Hope For Horses like the rest of us horse lovers. He was even asked to join Hope's board of directors. A few months later, he contacted me about Rowdy, a sixteen-year-old mini Shetland pony stallion that was in need of surgery to repair a broken hock on his left rear leg. An uncaring owner had stalled Rowdy with a large draft mare that kicked him repeatedly until he was rescued. John asked me for ideas about how to fundraise for Rowdy's surgery. We promoted the fundraiser by linking to it on our website and connected him with Deborah Sprague, the Windchill artist. She painted a fantastic picture of Rowdy and held a raffle online to raise money for his surgery. Raindance also offered to match the first five hundred dollars raised.

They raised more than two thousand dollars. "I can honestly say that if not for the heart and spirit of a little colt named Windchill, for the compassion and devotion of Jeff and Kathi Tucker, and for all the wonderful people who have come together at the Windchill Legacy website and forum, Rowdy might not have been saved," John wrote to us. "And I would likely be continuing along my ordinary life, completely oblivious to the needs of so many unwanted horses.

"Thank you, Windchill."

It's thrilling to see Windchill's legacy inspire others. A couple stopped by Raindance a few months after Windchill died to tell us they were building a barn at their place in Iron River, Wisconsin. They, too, would be accepting rescue horses. See what I mean? Windchill's influence continues. One step at a time.

Epilogue

Not a single day has passed since February 29, 2008, that I haven't thought about Windchill. I often wonder where he would be today had he lived. How big he would be now? Would he still have that cute personality the world fell in love with?

I learned so much from him in such a short time. The greatest lesson he taught me is that the simplest stories are often the most powerful. Perhaps in today's high-tech, fast-paced society it takes something simple to get through to us. A baby born in a manger. The smile of a child. A little colt who still had faith in people when he had every right to have none.

Possibly the best demonstration of how Windchill connected total strangers was the First Annual Windchill Legacy Barbeque, held at Raindance the summer after Windchill died. Several hundred people came that first year. It felt as if all who attended were lifelong friends. The usual discomfort of first meetings didn't exist. Hugs and laughter were immediate. It was one of the most amazing, humbling things I have experienced. Car after car arrived with excited folks who would jump out and tell us who they were from the online

Windchill forum. With each arrival, everyone cheered and there was another round of hugs.

These get-togethers have continued every summer, with an average of 100 to 125 people attending from the likes of New York, Arizona, Florida, Oregon, California, and Canada. A committee plans the entire event, from food and beverages to coordinating volunteers to help with parking, registration, and managing the silent auction. The auction has raised several thousand dollars for the Windchill Legacy.

I continue to hear from strangers who have just heard of Windchill. In addition to the thousands who learn of his story every year from our outreach to schools and senior citizen facilities, people still stumble across his story on the Internet. E-mails from people around the world continue to trickle in. Others discover the story on Facebook at the Legacy's page. A lady posted one day, "Hey, remember me—I'm the one who ordered Old Chicago pizzas for you [during the rescue]." I did remember and was happy to finally have someone to thank.

When I embarked on this book, I wanted the reader to finish it with renewed faith in the goodness of humanity. Despite the appearances of today's weary world, within most of us there is a strong desire to help others. Grown men would visit the farm to see "what all the fuss was about." Almost without fail, they grew silent at the sight of Windchill in his stall. A few moments later I would glance over to see tears streaming down their faces. These were big, tough guys. Guys who do construction or work for the county on the roads or in law enforcement. And there they stood—crying at what their fellow man had done to an innocent being. And there was Windchill—cranking his head around to see who his new friend was with those intensely bright eyes of his. It was so powerful. We would stand in silence for a while, then eventually we would give them their space and pretend to be preoccupied with something in the barn.

When Windchill died, there was such an enormous outpouring of sympathy via cards and e-mails, I sensed people needed to comfort one another. So despite suffering from pneumonia that left me barely able to sit up, I raced to get an online forum up and running for those who wanted to say goodbye to Windchill and talk to each other. With the help of a programmer friend, the forum was active within days of Windchill's death. The initial platform couldn't handle the volume of people, so my friend had to move it to a platform with more bandwidth built to handle hundreds of people at once.

This new forum also allowed me to step back as the gatekeeper to Windchill's online community. I could no longer handle the overwhelming intensity of emotions being thrown at me all at once. Yet I knew their pain. I was deep within it. In time I answered every single e-mail I ever received regarding Windchill.

Joining the thousands who signed his guestbook online every day were kids from around the country. Many of them learned about Windchill with daily updates at their schools. During the rescue, I answered the children's e-mails at night. I wanted to give them a response as soon as I could, so they knew people listened to them. When Windchill died, I wanted to write a goodbye note to them from Windchill. I realized hundreds, perhaps thousands, of children across the country were learning about death and the loss of a friend possibly for the first time. I felt it was important they see his death in a positive light. I wanted them to know their belief in Windchill made a difference.

> Dear littler people,
>
> I wanted to thank all of you for the cards and letters and pictures. I asked one of those that care for me to send you back my feelings, and he promised that he would.
>
> Your love and caring for me made me feel special, made me feel warm inside, and filled up a place in me that had been empty.

Sometimes it feels like big people don't hear what you say, doesn't it? I hope your big people do. They must if they let you send me all those pretty pictures. I lived someplace once where they didn't hear me, but then somebody did. They brought me to a warm place. They fed me. They held me like I hope your big people do you. They told me that they loved me. And then they showed me your words and your pictures, and I learned that kids like you see things just like me. So I was not alone. That made me very happy, which made me feel even warmer inside.

Thank you for telling me you loved me and making me feel so much better. I will always remember that you cared, and it will become a part of who I am deep in my heart. And you know what? Now that I know the words I can say them back to you: I love you too.

Your friend forever,
Windchill

As they grow, I hope Windchill's kids realize this story is proof one person can make a difference. One person went to check on a frozen colt. One person brought back another to load that colt in a trailer and bring it home. One more person helped unload the colt. One more gave us life-extending advice. Two more published a story on the front page of a newspaper that led to twenty-five thousand more people spreading the word through forums and websites that these people in the middle of nowhere were trying to save a little horse. One person read of our need for alfalfa hay and had it to us the next day. One person read of our trying to jury-rig warm socks to keep his legs warm and fired up her sewing machine. One person read of our coffee consumption and shipped us coffee. One person read we weren't eating well and shipped us pizza. Another person brought over casseroles. In the end all of these "one persons" made a world of difference to us and to Windchill.

Windchill's story shows us how, in this Internet age, we are no longer alone. One quickly accelerates to many, so no longer can any "one" of us use the excuse "but I'm only one person." I can't begin to say thanks enough to each of those people who changed Windchill's world. And mine. I will never forget them.

Time continues its endless march—often in directions we don't expect. I lost my son in November 2008. The suddenness of losing him inspired another mission for me, along with the rest of the family and friends of Jordan Lee Tucker: to spread the message to have your child's heart checked. Jordan was eighteen years and five days old when he passed away. He was a healthy athlete, honor student, and volunteer referee for a youth soccer league. One moment he was kidding with the family, fifteen minutes later he closed his eyes and never opened them again. His final words were a text message to a friend: "My heart is racing. Maybe I'm having a heart attack. LOL." Guess what? He was. That year was a painful journey into loss I hope to never have to travel again.

Another unexpected direction found Kathi and me deciding to part ways. We married the summer after the Windchill rescue. Windchill brought us together, but we learned that wasn't enough. Our dreams were just too different. I can't stress enough that if not for the amazing efforts of Kathi, Windchill's final moments on this earth would not have been the peaceful departure surrounded by love that he experienced. Those moments would have been much more horrific, and his story would never have seen the light of day. The tiny colt left to freeze to death in a northern Wisconsin pasture would have been just another silent victim of neglect.

As for me, I'll continue loving horses. Windchill forever changed my world. He changed how I view it. The world is a much smaller place now, since I've met so many good people from all over the country. I'm still searching for the same thing in my life as I think Windchill was in his: one more hello than goodbyes.

And just like Windchill, I believe.

Crisis in the Equine Industry

CAROLYN L. STULL, PHD

The number of unwanted horses in the United States has been estimated at well over one hundred thousand for the past few years. These horses may be old, be injured, exhibit dangerous behaviors, or not be trainable for their intended use. Or the owner may be financially or physically unable to care for the horse. Many of these unwanted and unmarketable horses would have been sent to slaughter facilities in the past, with their meat exported to other countries for human consumption. Due to public pressure in 2007, new federal regulations shut down equine slaughter plants in the United States. Thus the combination of slaughter plant closures, the economic depression initiated in 2008, along with rising feed and fuel costs have precipitated a dramatically depressed horse market with a much greater supply of horses than demand. As such, many owners can't even give their horses away to new homes.

The role of horses in society has transitioned over the last hundred years from one of work to pleasure. Or as some owners call them: "Pasture pets." However, when these pets become unwanted, they are not being afforded the facilities and adoption programs that are commonly provided for cats and dogs by taxpayer-funded municipal shelters in local communities. Instead, nonprofit equine rescue and sanctuary organizations in the United States have historically been responsible for providing both temporary and permanent care for relinquished horses, and many offer rehabilitation and adoption programs. In a nationwide survey published in 2010, it was estimated that there were approximately 326 nonprofit organizations in the United States that accept horses, but their total combined capacity was only 13,400 horses, well below the 100,000 horses believed to be unwanted (see K. E. Holcomb, C. L. Stull, and P. H. Kass, "Unwanted Horses: The Role of Nonprofit Equine Rescue and Sanctuary Organizations," *Journal of Animal Science* 88 [2010]: 4142–50, http://www.journalofanimalscience.org/content/88/12/4142). Many of these horses are compromised in their health and nutrition at the time of acceptance by these organizations. The body weight or condition of about 64 percent of the horses was described in the survey to be within the range of "thin to extremely emaciated," along with approximately half of the relinquished horses considered ill, injured, or lame.

Survey data collected on equine rescue and sanctuary organizations showed that funding and capacity are the limiting factors to their potential expansion to care for the current population of unwanted and neglected horses. This limited capacity may be due to a variety of factors, including low adoption rates and euthanasia policies. On an average, for every four horses relinquished to an organization, only three are adopted or sold to new owners. Few equine organizations practice wholesale euthanasia, such as many cat and dog municipal shelters do. This limits the number of horses over time accepted by the organizations. Funding is the greatest challenge to the continued operation of these facilities, with the maintenance costs of a relinquished horse averaging $3,648 per year.

These organizations are financially supported through personal funds and donations, and rely on volunteers for help. Effective education programs for responsible horse breeding and ownership may decrease the number of unwanted horses in the future. Donations, both private and corporate, will be the critical link in providing continual care by equine rescue and sanctuary organizations in order to safeguard the welfare on many unwanted horses within the United States.

How to Help

Organizations

The following organizations connect people who want to become involved in equine rescue and care. This is in no way to be considered a complete list, so please contact animal welfare organizations in your area also. I do not intend to officially endorse any of the following, but I know they serve as a good start for those who want to learn more about and help unwanted and/or neglected horses.

American Horse Defense Fund. http://ahdf.org/.
Equine Welfare Alliance. http://equinewelfarealliance.org/.
Horse Welfare Organizations. http://www.horse-welfare.org/.
The Windchill Legacy Ltd. http://www.thewindchilllegacy.org/.

Rescue Articles, Information, and Resources

American Association of Equine Producers (AAEP). "FAQs: Equine Cruelty, Abuse and Neglect." January 2012. http://www.aaep.org/images/files/AAEP%20FAQs%20Equine%20Abuse.pdf.

American Horse Defense Fund. "List of Horse Rescues." http://ahdf.org/rescue.htm.

Behind the Bit. "Equine Rescues: Which Ones Are Reputable?" February 22, 2008. http://www.behindthebitblog.com/2008/02/equine-rescues-which-ones-are-reputable.html.

The Foothills Focus. "Local Rescues Offer Animal Cruelty Prevention Tips." April 14, 2010. http://www.thefoothillsfocus.com/041410-horsecruelty.asp.

Helping Equines. "Listings of Horse Rescue Organizations." http://www.helpingequines.org/images/Helping_Equines_Rescue_List_08182007.pdf.

The Horse. "Finding a Reputable Rescue." November 9, 2010. http://cs.thehorse.com/blogs/horses-and-the-law/archive/2010/11/09/finding-a-reputable-rescue.aspx.

Horse Channel. "Rescue Organizations." http://www.horsechannel.com/horse-resources/rescue-organizations.aspx.

The Real Owner. "What to Do When You Suspect Animal Abuse." March 8, 2010. http://therealowner.com/adoption-rescue/what-to-do-when-you-suspect-animal-abuse/.

Whispering Way Natural Horsemanship. "Find a Horse Rescue Near You!" http://www.naturalhorsetraining.com/horserescues.html.

Acknowledgments

When the Windchill rescue was occurring, I tried at the time to thank everybody on the blog and website. What I quickly found out was that there were more people to thank then there was time available to thank them. I had to acknowledge the generosity of our fellow humans in a general way and thus had to thank the world. And so I will thank a few people here by name, but I acknowledge in a huge way that none of what you just read would have been possible without the generous caring and outpouring of support that came from so many. To all of you, thank you from the bottom of my heart.

Thank you, Team Windchill—as the volunteers who sat around the clock with him and the lift crew came to be known. Your unwavering support and caring for Windchill made his life and our lives so much better.

Thank you, Dr. Carolyn L. Stull and the University of California–Davis. Your advice and steadfast support despite pressure to not assist us was both crucial and reassuring. Your patience and, in the end, your sympathy will never be forgotten.

Thank you to the media. You taught me events can be more than just a story, and though you are hidden behind the need for objectivity in your reporting, I learned you have a heart.

Thank you, Judith Munson. Judith volunteered during the Windchill rescue to help respond to the constant bombardment of e-mails and media requests (a request I wish I hadn't declined in hindsight!), and I turned to her when the time came to organize my notes into a book. Judith's expertise helped turn my writing from snippets into organization—not a small task.

And lastly, thank you to the world that responded to a little being's need with a generosity that was truly humbling. Your prayers, donations, gifts, visits, and positive energy meant everything to us. You connected with the spirit of a nine-month-old colt whose faith and belief eliminated borders, making the world a smaller place, and teaching us that strangers are just friends we haven't met yet.